Children and the Dark Side of Human Experience

D0837404

James Garbarino

Children and the Dark Side of Human Experience

Confronting Global Realities and Rethinking Child Development

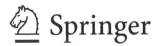 Springer

James Garbarino
Loyola University
Chicago, IL
USA

ISBN: 978-0-387-75625-7   e-ISBN: 978-0-387-75626-4
DOI: 10.1007/978-0-387-75626-4

Library of Congress Control Number: 2008920254

Printed on acid-free paper

9 8 7 6 5 4 3 2 1

springer.com

For Urie Bronfenbrenner (1917–2005)
Friend, mentor, and colleague

Contents

Introduction

And they were bringing children to Him so that He might touch them; and the disciples rebuked them. But when Jesus saw this, He was indignant and said to them, "Permit the children to come to Me; do not hinder them; for the kingdom of God belongs to such as these."

—Mark, 10:13–14

I began writing this book during a trip to Japan in January 2002. While in the country I started reading anthropologist Ruth Benedict's classic analysis of Japanese society and culture, *The Sword and the Chrysanthemum*. Written at the close of World War II to help the American government plan for defeating the Japanese war machine and dealing with a defeated nation, Benedict wrote several things that struck home as I began my own work a half century later. For one thing, as she reviewed indigenous Japanese social analyses she cautioned, "They were amazingly frank. Of course they did not present the whole picture. No people does. A Japanese who writes about Japan passes over really crucial things which are as familiar to him and as invisible as the air he breathes. So do Americans when they write about America" (p. 7). That is part of the challenge I faced, to see what is invisible in front of our eyes.

The German poet Goethe spoke of this when he wrote:

"What is most difficult of all?
That which you think is easiest,
To see what is before your eyes."

Benedict spoke of this too. She wrote, "Writers of every nation have tried to give an account of themselves. But it is not easy. The lenses through which any nation looks at life are not the ones another nation uses. It is hard to be conscious of the eyes through which one looks" (p. 14).

I attach great importance to my visits with children in societies around the world as well as in my native United States. But as important to me as my experiences were, I must always remember that I was a visitor to these children and their lives. I was a visitor in the desperately poor shanty towns of Brazil, in the grim Vietnamese detention camps in Hong Kong, in the arid desert of Sudan, in the desperate street battles between Israelis and Palestinians, and even to the angry young men on death row and the scared children coping with living in Chicago neighborhoods plagued with gang violence. But my status as an outsider in these worlds is not an automatic disqualification. In fact, it can be the start of insight.

It is said that comparison is essential for understanding. Assuming a fish could describe anything, how could a fish describe water if it had not known air? I have learned that there is a special risk and a special opportunity to be found in being a stranger in a strange land. Sometimes a foreigner sees things that a native does not. The risk is that the foreigner will be taken in by superficial illusions and miss the deeper reality. This happened to the great anthropologist Margaret Mead, for example, in her early field work among the Polynesian peoples of the South Pacific. It became clear in later years that "the natives" were messing with her head, and deliberately filling it with exaggerations and outright fabrications.

When I traveled to China in 1981, I heard the adage (attributed to a Jesuit priest of the eighteenth century) that "If you visit China for a week you know enough to write a letter about it. If you stay for a month you know enough to write an article. If you stay a year you know enough to write a book. But if you stay longer than a year you know enough to write nothing at all." My brief trips to extreme situations around the world lay me open to the wisdom of that observation. I know that.

Perhaps I should be wise enough to write nothing, but I cannot remain silent because there is special value to the foreigner's observations. Perhaps it is for this reason that many of the most incisive and insightful analyses of America, for example, have been done by foreigners, with the nineteenth century Frenchman de Tocqueville's, *Democracy in America* being the best known example. I don't claim to be able to fill de Tocqueville's shoes, but with 30 years of studying child and youth development behind me (but under my belt) I feel I do have something to contribute.

As I began this book I was setting out to translate my experiences into a set of lessons learned about how to understand and protect the human rights of children and youth in extreme situations. I was seeking to formulate some principles about resilience and coping amidst trauma, exploitation, danger, and social toxicity. I was trying to bring my spiritual perspective to the world of children living on the dark side of human experience. I learned that doing the right thing for and about kids in extreme situations is neither simple nor easy, not intellectually, not emotionally.

In life in general, it may be hard to recognize danger and the pathways to safety unless you have special tools and guidance. For example, most of us are not well-equipped or -positioned to monitor the quality of the water we drink. It requires specialized knowledge and equipment to assess the presence and risks posed by water-borne toxins. Understanding and protecting the human rights of children makes the same demands. The sources and risks of social and psychological toxicity in the lives of children are not always obvious or easily mastered, particularly if the goal is more than to simply document suffering and damage. I have been at this task of understanding children at risk for more than three decades, and I have learned some important lessons. The first one is that kids are spiritual beings; they crave meaning in their lives.

We know that children are physical beings. As such they have physical needs. Deprive them of essential nutrients, calories, and vitamins and their physical development is warped. They can even die if the deprivation becomes serious enough.

By the same token, we know that children are psychological beings. They have psychological needs. For example, deprive them of acceptance and their development is likely to warp. This is the truth underlying anthropologist Ronald Rohner's classic work on rejection. Rohner studied 118 cultures around the world and found that in each culture, kids who are rejected turn out badly, so much so that Rohner called rejection a "psychological malignancy."

By the same token, kids have spiritual needs. Foremost among these spiritual needs is the need to know you live in a meaningful universe, that there is something more than the material experience of your life. This is not simply a matter of religion, however.

Some religious experiences do not meet spiritual needs very well; some people meet their spiritual needs outside the structures of organized religion. Wherever it is that they find their spiritual sustenance, however, one truth is clear: Children need to grow up with a sense that they have a positive place in the universe, that there is a force of loving acceptance that infuses and supports their lives, and that there is something more to life than the material experience of it. They need this particularly as they move from childhood into adolescence. It is this lesson that is so fundamental to what I have learned about and from kids in extreme situations around the world that I can only introduce it here, with the promise that I will return to it again and again in the chapters to follow.

I've met and interviewed many parents over the last 25 years, in the United States and around the world, and almost every single one of them wants the best for themselves and their child. Their intentions are generally good. And I have spoken with scores of professionals—teachers, social workers, physicians, counselors, nurses, and therapists—and each of them wants the best for kids. And I have met and spoken with many public officials and political leaders—at the White House, in Congress, at the United Nations, in state houses, and in conference centers around the country and the world. And mostly they too want things to be better for kids.

I speak particularly to my fellow Americans when I say this, but say it I must: Translating good intentions into effective action and relationships in the world in general, and in raising the next generation to fulfill those positive aspirations is difficult. The complexity of human development is such that good intentions are insufficient. As one wag put it: "You can change the world … but unless you know what you are doing, please don't!" How do we move beyond American good intentions, particularly when we are talking about kids in extreme situations?

First, we must do something that we as Americans are generally loathe to do. We must look deeply and from a well-grounded theoretical foundation. We must avoid simply plunging into action, and instead take the time to look at things through a theoretical lens. Americans like simplicity and action. Reality often does not oblige. German psychologist Kurt Lewin tried to bridge this gap when he wrote, "There is nothing so practical as a good theory."

It sounds almost un-American to say this. We like action. We want just the facts. Theory and depth do not come naturally to us. We like to have what we need to know in a one-page letter or even a brief e-mail. As a result, we sometimes blunder into disasters because our naïve and simplistic view of things crashes into reality in all its complexity. A case in point is the 2003 war in Iraq, which looked at first like a simple military campaign to overthrow a dictator, but became a complex morass of competing claims and suffering. Looking back at it in 2008, the folly of the invasion is apparent to all but the most ideologically or self-interestedly blinded.

To get beyond the shallow and misleadingly obvious requires something more, not just for a small group of elite academic intellectuals, but for all of us. It requires that we dig deeper than the sound bite. It is one thing to respond emotionally to the sights and sounds of hungry refugee children shivering with cold in an Afghan refugee camp or a bunker in a Bosnian war zone, or even a first grader in a Chicago public school traumatized by gang violence. It is quite another to think deeply and respond in an informed way to these children—and even more importantly, the angry, troubled, and sometimes dangerous teenagers they may become.

When it comes to matters of human development, simplicity is the exception rather than the rule. For our actions to be effective they must be grounded in a deeper understanding. Child development research teaches us that children are not just short adults. They think and feel in ways that are different from the ways adults think and feel, and these develop over time. For example, most preschool children have difficulty understanding that if you pour a liquid from a short fat container into a tall thin one the two containers hold the same amount of liquid. Most preschool children think the thin tall container has more liquid in it, even though they have seen you pour it from the short fat one. This ability to "conserve" volume isn't reliably present in most children until they are 8 years old. Very few adults lack this ability to understand that the volume of a liquid doesn't change when you move it from one vessel to another.

By the same token, many adolescents have trouble recognizing the emotions conveyed by different facial expressions. When shown faces that adults can reliably identify as expressing fear, many adolescents think they are seeing shock or anger. Why? It seems to reflect the fact that the part of the brain that processes this information is still immature in young adolescents.

Children under the age of 10 seem to be more vulnerable to being traumatized when exposed to awful events than teenagers and adults. One study found that the same events that produced psychological symptoms of trauma (what is commonly called posttraumatic stress disorder) in 56% of kids 10 and younger only produced those symptoms in 18% of teenagers and adults. This finding serves to reinforce the point that knowing child development is an important resource to understanding the complex interplay of forces that influence the lives and deaths of children and youth.

To see the whole picture we must do more than have "the facts." We must develop in ourselves the greatest possible creative intuition and insight. With that intuition and insight we are capable of what it takes to meet the challenge of understanding children so that we can evaluate and meet the threats that undermine development. What it takes is a mix of insightful analysis of a child's behavior, coupled with the ability to feel and see things as they see and feel them. I call this double ability "intelligent empathy"—being able to understand a child's inner life through a mix of knowledge about child development and appreciation for how life feels to a specific child or group of children.

To accomplish this, adults need to develop at least two kinds of creative insight in their relationships with children. The first, and most common, is when someone knows what is going on inside a particular child because of a special relationship with that child. My mentor, psychologist Urie Bronfenbrenner, often said that the key to good child development is the child having at least one adult who is crazy about that child, someone who believes the sun rises and sets in the eyes of that child. This commitment is intensely individualized.

This is the basis for the kind of insight parents develop most of the time from living with their child. Mom says, "Something's going on with Tommy today. I just know something's wrong." Dad replies, "I noticed it too. Maybe something happened at school today." Parents know a child in depth, in detail, and in context. This knowledge is specific to a particular child and may not apply to all children.

This first kind of insight is not enough, particularly for dealing with someone else's children, particularly if those children are faced with extreme situations. The second kind of insight is more general. It is the ability to understand children in general, being able to understand a child even without having a long-standing special relationship with that child.

This is what teachers and other child development professionals count on in their work. A 6-year-old plays with puppets as his therapist watches the melodrama that unfolds between the big bear and the little bear. The therapist says to the child, "I think you are angry at your Dad because you think he is going to leave you the way he left your Mom." She says this in light of what she has just seen, because of what she knows about children. It flows from the fact that she has practiced listening to children and she has had good training, education, and supervision by her professional elders.

This second kind of insight takes hard work, study, and emotional commitment on the part of the adult. It results from firmly believing that what children do and say make sense if approached from the child's point of view. It comes from looking anew—with this new insight into the meaning of what children do and say—at the dinner table, in the car, on the playground, getting ready for bed, in the classroom, in the therapist's office.

Psychoanalyst Bruno Bettelheim and psychiatrist Alvin Rosenfeld called this looking anew without blinders "the art of the obvious." Once you understand deeply, the child's previously "crazy" or "meaningless" behavior becomes clearer as to its purpose and its relationship to the child's experience and development. It's worth returning to how the German poet Goethe captured this difficulty when he wrote, "What is most difficult? That which you think is easiest, to see what is before your eyes."

The art of the obvious takes a willingness to open yourself to children, to use your own experience as a way to make contact with them. It takes a commitment to put aside judgment in favor of acceptance, substitute knowledge of child development for bias and myth, and be willing to open yourself to the emotional life of the child rather than experiencing everything from an adult point of view. When all of this comes together I call it intelligent empathy. It is a starting point; but is not enough in and of itself.

We need a perspective on human development that begins with the realization that there are few hard and fast simple rules about how human beings develop; complexity is the rule rather than the exception. Where I come from intellectually we call this an "ecological perspective" on human development. It means that when you look at research on how people develop from infancy to old age you find that rarely, if ever, is there a simple cause–effect relationship that works the same way for all people in every situation. Rather, when you open your eyes to it you find that the process of cause and effect depends upon the whole picture of who the individual is and where the phenomena are occurring.

If we ask, "does X cause Y?" the best scientific answer is almost always "it depends." It depends upon:

- Gender. (The amount of infant babbling predicts childhood IQ in girls but not boys.)
- Temperament—the particular emotional package brought into the world by a child. (About 10% of children are born with a temperamental proneness to becoming "shy," but this predisposition can be overcome with strong, support- ive, and long-term intervention.)
- Age. (On average, teenagers can understand abstract concepts of time better than children.)
- Neighborhood. (Although in some neighborhoods 60% of 10 year olds with a chronic pattern of aggression, acting out and violating the rights of others, end up as serious violent delinquents, in other neighborhoods the figure is only 15%.)
- Culture (Native Hawaiians see the goal of child rearing as producing an interde- pendent person, whereas most Americans seek to create rugged individualists. As a result, singling children out for special attention in classrooms works well for most American children but not most Hawaiian children, because for the latter being separated from the group is shameful rather than a source of pride.)

This ecological perspective is frustrating: We all would prefer a simple "yes or no" to the question "does X cause Y?" But reality is not obliging on this score. One important corollary of our ecological perspective is the fact that generally it is the accumulation of risks and assets in a child's life that tells the story, not the presence or absence of any one negative or positive influence.

Psychologist Mavis Hetherington's book, *For Better and For Worse: Children of Divorce*, provides an illuminating example. Her decades of research reveal that most kids overcome the challenge of living with divorce in childhood—perhaps 75%—but a significant minority—the other 25%—do experience deep troubles. What influences who will manage the challenge and who will not? It is mostly the extent to which children have to cope with divorce in addition to other risk factors inside and around them.

Most children can live with one major risk factor; few can handle a mountain of them. Getting from a generalized "it depends" to a more specific assessment of the likely fate of any child lies in accounting for all the elements of accumulated risk factors, developmental assets, and temperament to determine the odds of success or failure. Does divorce produce long-lasting negative effects? As always, the answer is "it depends." That's always the answer in general, but once we know what else a particular child is facing—poverty? drug abuse in a parent? child abuse? racism? too many siblings?—we can move closer to "yes, probably" or "no, probably not." One important influence on these contingencies is always the temperament of the child.

Each person offers a distinctive emotional package, a temperament. Each child shows up in the world with a different package of characteristics. Some are more sensitive; others are less so. Some are very active; some are lethargic. Why are these differences important? For one thing, they affect how much and in what direction the world around them will influence how they think and feel about things.

What one person can tolerate another will experience as highly destructive. What will be overwhelming to one of us will be a minor inconvenience to another. Knowing a child's temperament goes a long way toward knowing how vulnerable that child will be to the world, particularly to extreme situations. Chess and Thomas' classic research on temperament reported that although about 70% of "difficult" babies evidenced serious adjustment problems by elementary school, the figure was only 10% for "easy" babies.

Standing against the accumulation of risk are the number of developmental assets in a child's life and the components of resilience. Research conducted by the Search Institute has identified 40 developmental assets—positive characteristics of family, school, neighborhood, peers, culture, and belief systems. As these assets accumulate, the likelihood that a child or adolescent will be engaged in antisocial violence declines; for example, from 61% for kids with 0–10 assets, to 6% for kids with 31–40. Asset accumulation predicts resilient response to stress and challenge.

Although it is defined in numerous ways, resilience generally refers to an individual's ability to stand up to adverse experiences, avoid long-term negative effects, or otherwise overcome developmental threats. Every one knows someone whose life is a testament to resilience. The concept of resilience rests on the research finding that although there is a correlation between specific negative experiences and explicit negative outcomes, in most situations a majority (perhaps 60%–80%) of children and youth will not display that negative outcome.

All of us have some capacity to deal with adversity, but some of us have more than others and are thus more resilient, whereas others are more vulnerable in difficult times. However, some of us face relatively easy lives, whereas others face mountains of difficulty with few allies and resources. In every situation there is some room for us to act better or worse; how we respond is a measure of our character. All of this is clarified and explicated in the chapters of this book, where we look directly at children in specific extreme situations. However, a few more words are in order here on the topic of resilience.

Resilience is not absolute. Virtually every kid has a breaking point or an upper limit on stress absorption capacity. Kids are malleable rather than resilient, in the sense that each threat costs them something. What is more, in some environments virtually all youth demonstrate negative effects of highly stressful and threatening environments. For example, in his Chicago data psychologist Patrick Tolan looked at the impact of overwhelming risk accumulation. He measured resilience at age 15 as managing for a 2-year period being neither more than one grade level behind in school, nor having sufficient mental health problems that warrant professional intervention. His findings? None of the minority, adolescent males facing a combination of highly dangerous and threatening low-income neighborhoods coupled with low-resource/high-stress families was resilient (which is not to say that they never recovered and got back on track; some did).

What is more, resilience in gross terms may obscure real costs to the individual. Some people manage to avoid succumbing to the risk of social failure as defined by poverty and criminality, but nonetheless experience real harm in the form of diminished capacity for successful intimate relationships. Even apparent social success—performing well in the job market, avoiding criminal activity, and creating a family—may obscure some of the costs of being resilient in a socially toxic environment, such as that faced by millions of youth.

The inner lives of these individuals may be fraught with emotional damage, for example, to self-esteem and intimacy. Although resilient in social terms, these individuals may be severely wounded souls. In a sense, this may parallel what has long been evident in comparing the resilience of boys with that of girls. Traditionally, boys who succumb to the accumulation of risk have long been prone to act out in explicitly antisocial behavior (juvenile delinquency), whereas girls have been more likely to respond with internalized symptoms of distress. Does this mean girls are more resilient than boys? A simple accounting of social success variables might lead us to think so. However, if we take into account the full range of manifestations of harm we see that such an answer is wrong. Kids adapt, for better and for worse, and they do so in counterpoint to the healthiness of the social environments in which they live.

Just as physical poisons in the environment have an effect on our physical health, psychological and cultural toxins in the social environment influence our mental and spiritual well-being. I offer the term "social toxicity" as a parallel concept to physical toxicity as a threat to human well-being and survival, and I return to it in detail in a later chapter. However, throughout my focus is always on the human rights of children, rights that flow directly from my spiritual orientation. Why is this so important? I think its importance flows in part from the fact that this understanding of a higher purpose and power to life beyond the material is the bedrock upon which a belief in human rights is founded. In this I am with those like Emory University Law Professor Michael Perry, who realize that without God (in whatever form one understands that concept) there is no appeal beyond "interest," and thus no basis for asserting the kind of absolute commitments upon which concepts like "the inherent dignity of the human person" must rest. *Human rights exist because human beings are "God's children," and therefore other human beings and institutions are not entitled to violate that privileged status.*

My goal always is to see in the particulars of each child's situation a greater understanding of the human condition, a broader recognition of what it means to be human, and a clearer picture of what is required of us to heal the wounds of kids in life-and-death situations. In every situation I always ask, "What lessons can we learn about the human rights of children and how we can preserve and support those rights?" With this in mind, let us begin this journey to the dark side of human experience so that we may understand and ultimately protect the children who live there.

Chapter 1
How Can We Think About Children Confronting the Dark Side of Human Experience?

How do we know what we need to know about the human rights of children and youth? I start from a belief that there are three principal paths to understanding: science and humanities, subjective human studies, and soul searching. Each is a way of trying to know, a process rather than an event. A complete understanding requires all three: Matters of life and death demand it.

Let me give an example of how these three ways of knowing coexist in the real world, an example that mirrors the issues we face in life as a whole. Consider children playing a game—perhaps a group of 10 year olds playing soccer. The outcome of the game hinges on the skill of the players as well as random variations in success (and the premise of a fair and competent referee, of course). So where do the three ways of knowing come into the game?

The science of the game hinges on the fact that the link between the skill of the players and the outcome of the game is neither fixed nor completely random. In this, the case mirrors human life in many important aspects. For example, the odds that a human being will live to be 80 years old are known at birth based upon gender, social class, time, and place. The odds are particularly good if you are a female born in the twenty-first century in a middle-class family living in affluent First World country and rather poor if you are a female born in a destitute family living in a village in Bangladesh or some other Third World country. But odds only apply to large numbers of multiple events and never completely account for outcome.

From a subjective human studies perspective, the soccer game (like each of our lives) is about each contestant's specific experience and what it means to that individual. Some kids are more coordinated than others, but whether or not this translates into a goal or a winning game is not known in advance.

The other biographical dimension of the game lies in the fact that the significance of the playing and whether or not you win the game depends upon who you are as an individual. Thus, for a child with parents who seek their own gratification in their child's athletic performance, for a child of low self-esteem or for one with intense emotional investment in being a winner, the stakes are high. For another child the result may be trivial in comparison with the pleasure of playing the game and being part of a team.

Here too, the game mirrors human life on Earth. Each of us has a personal story. These stories are particular to our "luck" from day to day and year to year, our talents

and abilities, how our environment welcomes or rejects them, and how we respond
to these events to create our emergent stories. For example, some children in both
the affluent First World and the destitute Third World defy the statistical odds of
their situation: Some American kids die in the first year of life; some Bangladeshi
kids live to be 90. What is more, among both children and 90 year olds in every
society there are variations in the perceived quality and meaning of their lives. Some
poor kids experience a story of happy, content meaningfulness, whereas some rich
kids tell a story of sadness, despair, and nihilism. Whatever it is, each individual's
story is a unique expression of how he or she encounters and experiences life.

What about soul searching? From a deep perspective, the soccer game is at best
an amusing and entertaining diversion. Trophies or other prizes to be won are minor
matters. Although in general life may be more comfortable with success on the
playing field, soul searching reveals that if the process of obtaining or having any
form of worldly success distracts from enlightenment and love, then it is a dangerous delusion.

It's only a game, after all, *as is everything material that does not nourish the
spiritual*. Once again, this mirrors human life in general. From the perspective of
spirit, how long you live is not the issue, but always how well you live. I thought of
this in October 2002, when I was asked to deliver a talk at a church in Virginia at
the time the Beltway Sniper was at large—shooting at random people in the area of
the church.

I recall the conference organizers' concerns that attendance would be down
because of people's fears of going out in public and thus exposing themselves to
the shooter. I remember the palpable anxiety as my host and his family exited their
minivan and walked from the parking lot to the church building. As I stood at the
pulpit I spoke of the irony of this situation. Certainly one of the core beliefs of
Christianity is that you must always be ready for death by living a life of faith. Jesus
spoke of this, saying, "I am the resurrection and the life. Those who believe in me,
even though they die, will live" (John 11:25).

It is a testament to the difficulty of living completely in congruence with our
spiritual beliefs that the many Christians attending the conference found it impossible to live as their faith instructed them to do. Living life guided by the spirit is
easy in the abstract, but difficult in the reality of day-to-day life.

The issue is always how you live the time you have. In the fall of 2005, two
deaths occurred in my social world within the space of one week's time. The first
was my 88-year-old mentor, Urie Bronfenbrenner, who died after a life of enormous worldly accomplishment and family proliferation (five children, 16 grandchildren, and two great grandchildren). The second was a 10-year-old boy in my
church who died after living most of his life with cancer. To all who knew him, the
little boy's life was completely fulfilled spiritually, even though it was grievously
abbreviated as a biography and was a physical catastrophe in scientific, objective
terms.

In the eternal world of the spirit, our time on Earth is a very minor matter, made
significant only by virtue of the fact that it affects our opportunities to engage the
universe and progress toward enlightenment. By all accounts, the little boy with

cancer lived a very spiritually efficient life in the sense that he achieved a rare level of consciousness and closeness to God in the few years of life on Earth available to him. No one would invite cancer into the life of a child just to create the opportunity for spiritual growth and consciousness, of course, but there is no denying that ultimately it is the spiritual accomplishments of living that matter most.

Having made the three forms of knowing concrete through an example, let me return to each in a more elaborated way, as a preparation for exploring how each affects the way we approach the issue of human rights for kids. Science and humanities are the domains of academics. Here we find the efforts of scientists and humanists. The former (both physical and social scientists) seek to demonstrate the objective empirical realities of human behavior and growth; the latter look for patterns in culture and history by analyzing literature and other human documents.

The goal of scientists is to document empirical patterns, statistical relationships, and predictive and verifiable hypotheses concerning the objective features of human development. Humanists seek to tease larger patterns of meaning out of documents—themes in history, literature, philosophy, and art.

Whether scientists or humanists, this is the predominant discourse in academic pursuit and policy making. It is the world of "on average" and "in general" and "on the whole" and "most" and "few" and "many." Both science and humanities have at their core a set of rules and principles to govern the pursuit of knowledge and its communication with others. In this sense both are "objective." This is not to say that biases don't creep into the process. They do. But the intellectual beauty of science and humanities is that there are well-established tactics and strategies for exposing and disposing of these infringements upon the fundamental commitment to objectivity when they are detected.

But although science and the humanities map the large-scale psychological, sociological, biological, cultural, and demographic terrain of human development, this alone does not lead us to the end of the journey. Set within this conception of life is the individual experience of being human, which inescapably leads us to a second methodology, the study of subjectivity in what some scholars have called human studies.

Human studies is the study of the unique meaning that individuals recognize in themselves, and the processes and strategies for communicating that meaning to others, albeit inadequately. There are an enormous number of specific influences on any single individual human being, influences that interact and accumulate to produce very different end results. Therefore, no two human beings share exactly the same life pathway; no two of us have exactly the same autobiography.

There are general commonalities, to be sure, and these are the object of study by science and humanities—for example, in a branch of psychology called life span development. Also, there are points of perfect intersection between separate lives, the points at which two individuals recognize that despite the myriad of differences that differentiate them as people there is a point of complete correspondence.

Nonetheless, subjective human studies recognizes that each individual life is unique in the experiencing of it. It asks us to try to walk miles in the shoes of another human being, although even as it asks us to adopt this strategy for feeling what the other feels—empathy—it recognizes that whatever we learn will be intrinsically and inevitably incomplete and approximate. This differentiates human studies from science and humanities, in which precision rules.

Subjective human studies demands that we allow room for a process that moves beyond the constraints of a purely academic focus on objectivity and verification. It demands that we allow for subjective information to become a valid vehicle for understanding developmental issues. Human studies focuses on the narrative accounts of subjective experience, on life stories, on autobiography.

It's about discovering and assessing the meaning of human experience as it is lived and understood by a specific individual. It's about human beings in their singularity as represented through the stories these human beings employ to make sense of themselves as individuals (and as members of groups). Human studies is the documentation of identity: It is each of us telling the story of his or her life. It's the study of biography.

Human studies seeks to illuminate subjectivity while acknowledging that any such effort can only be partial, no matter how long we work at it or how smart we are. It recognizes that no matter how good the story, how poignant and evocative the language of that story, and how diligent the listener's efforts, there is always loss of validity from the teller of the story to the listener. What we learn from the creating and telling of our life stories advances our understanding of the human experience, but it too is incomplete.

In other words, empathy is never complete. In human studies you can never know exactly what I am experiencing, unlike science, in which when I say the temperature of this liquid is 45 °F you can know exactly what that means and exactly replicate my data. Philosophers of science have called this phenomenon of you knowing what I know (and I knowing what you know) inter-subjective transmissibility.

All human communication is ultimately imperfect, thus inter-subjective transmissibility is always and inevitably partial and incomplete. Nevertheless, even were it complete, it would not be the whole human story, because human beings are more than the story of moving their bodies around on the planet Earth. Human beings are spiritual beings, and this requires yet another kind of knowing.

This third form of human study is soul searching. Here the goal is to make and sustain contact with human spiritual realities beyond the facts of physical experience, and even the individual's subjective account. Like science and humanities, there is a defining methodology to soul searching.

What is this method? It is contemplation, meditation, and prayer. It is what Zen Buddhists like Thich Nhat Hanh call mindfulness, the practice of paying attention to reality in the present moment. It is to sit quietly for a long time and focus your attention—perhaps through observing your breathing or through meditative prayer. The evidence is clear that if you follow this methodology you will reach approximately the same conclusions. In this sense, then, science and humanities share with soul searching the goal of documenting and illuminating common realities, whereas human studies seeks to document and illuminate particular realities.

In the case of soul searching, these common and objective conclusions find expression in statements such as: "There is more to life than the material experience of it," "Love is the fundamental imperative of the universe," and "Peace comes from caring without attachment and desire." As in the case with science and humanities, the particulars of what exactly this means in day-to-day life are sometimes and somewhat ambiguous and open to dispute.

From this perspective, religion is the intellectual and social infrastructure created to house and promote these three basic findings. Thus, each religion has its own take on these primary data—part of what the Jesuits I pray with mean by the expression "finding God in everything and everyone," and why they are so interested in finding spiritual truths and realities in every culture they encounter. What is more, some individuals discover these data without the benefits (or obstacles) of any specific religion, as long as they follow the method.

Apply the method and you reach the three basic data of soul searching, just as if you embrace the methodology of science and direct your attention to human biology you almost inevitably come to the conclusion that the current form of human bodies is the product of evolution—despite the claims of creationism or intelligent design. Similarly, whether you are the Christians' St. Ignatius of Loyola or St. Clare of Assisi, or the Buddhists' Thich Nhat Hanh or the Dalai Lama, the common method leads to the same essential results, although how you express these truths and what implications you draw for day-to-day living in the specific cultural and historical context of your life may vary.

Some Native American cultures speak of "soul traveling" as a way to integrate the experience of body/mind/brain/soul. Christian, Jewish, and Muslim mystics see the path in prayer. Buddhists and Hindus speak of insight meditation. This approach starts from the reality of human beings as spiritual beings having a physical experience, and proceeds from there. Does anything in human experience really mean anything beyond what individuals, groups, and cultures say it means? Is there anything more than psychology, biology, sociology, and anthropology on the one hand, and history and literature on the other? Without soul searching, the answer is no. With soul searching the answer is yes. As documented by Mario Beuegard and Denyse D'leary in their book *The Spiritual Brain*, there is a consciousness beyond the sum total of the physical biology of the human brain, a reality beyond the material.

If we do not recognize the spiritual realities underlying the literary realities of narrative accounts and the statistical descriptions of empirical realities of the social and physical sciences there is only one empirical reality—"You are born. You live. You die."—and only two basic narrative accounts—"I am born. I have a nice day. Then I die." or "I am born. My life sucks. Then I die."

Only soul searching can expand these stories by integrating them into the eternal realities of spirituality. Buddhism and Christianity offer elaborate world views that transcend the experience of conventional life and place the individual in the realm of the timeless, where oneness with the universe becomes obvious. You can't go there without this spiritual practice (but limiting yourself to the theology and practice of conventional religion may not take you there either).

Human beings are spiritual beings and thus have spiritual needs. No simply material conception of human identity will suffice. This is a vitally important recognition for understanding the quality of the world outside our front door; and this is very different from speaking about religion. The relationship between religion and spirituality is not simple. There are those who are religious but not spiritual, and vice versa. To recognize our spiritual needs is to recognize that we have a fundamental need to know we live in a meaningful universe, that there is something more to our lives than the material experience of those lives.

This brings us to the issue of human rights. Human rights derive not from some legal formulation, but from a core attitude toward human life and experience. One way to understand this is to explore the difference between sentimentality and compassion. I grew up in a very sentimental household, particularly when it came to animals. My mother was the sort who would root for the lions when it came down to a battle between the Christians and the lions. In a Western movie her concern was not for the cowboys and Indians, but for their horses. It took me quite a long time to see something beyond the significance of this sentimental rooting for the pathetic. It took the teaching of a great spiritual guide.

Tibet's Dalai Lama is a world leader in teaching about compassion. One of his most important lessons is that "true compassion is not just an emotional response, but a firm commitment founded on reason." It is easy to feel sympathy for the victims of violence; human decency demands it. But it is much more difficult to feel true compassion for our enemies; unshakable understanding of how violence and rage arise in human beings, understanding that endures the bad actions of those human beings. I have confronted this difficulty often in my work as an expert witness in murder trials, in which compassion is often in short supply.

This book brings the lessons of science, human studies, and soul searching to the topic of protecting the human rights of children facing the dark side of human experience. Admittedly, these kids live in situations that are alien to most readers: war zones, refugee camps, prisons, and the slums of Third World countries. Few Americans are familiar with these places; fewer still have been there.

Nonetheless, what happens in these places and to these children and teenagers who are growing up there matters to us all for two reasons. First, because we can learn important lessons from these places and kids that can help us manage our own complicated lives and situations. Second, because the world is a more connected place than it once was, and what happens anywhere and with anyone can affect what happens here, to us. If 9/11 taught us anything, it should have taught us that.

An Islamic religious fanatic with a grudge against American policy in the Middle East can bring down tall buildings and hold your entire society hostage to fear. An angry child in a refugee camp far away can become a vengeful terrorist intent upon blowing up you and your loved ones. The abused child who becomes the violent criminal may confront you in a dark alley some time. The poor sick child in China may spread a disease that you get in North America. The child living in poverty in Central America may make his way across the border to live in your city, go to your schools, and use your health care services. The war far away may come home to you, as a terrorist attacks your city.

But there is more. There is the simple moral obligation that each of us has to our fellow human beings. Every religion and ethical system in the world that is worth respecting contains at its core the insistence that we are one people. I learned this in Sunday school as a child: Jesus echoed Moses when he said, "Love thy neighbor as thyself." I learned it anew every time I participated as an adult in a spiritual retreat or read a book on ethics, whatever the religious tradition. I learned it in elementary school when we memorized the words of the eighteenth century English poet John Donne, "No Man is an island/no man stands alone." With this as a foundation we go forward with this moral imperative, to explore the human rights of children with fealty to our commitment to use all three ways of knowing to make sense of life on the dark side of human experience through understanding the human rights of children and how to protect them.

Chapter 2
The Right to Feel Safe: Trauma and Recovery

... to come face to face with human vulnerability in the natural world and with the capacity for evil in human nature.

—Susan Sgroi

Of all the human rights of children perhaps the most important is the right to be safe. As we shall see in later chapters, this right is often a matter of physical safety—being spared mutilation, starvation, or murder, for example. But from the perspective of child development, some of the most important threats to the child's right to be safe come in the form of traumatic experiences, experiences that threaten the development of heart and mind.

The word "trauma" has entered into common usage in America. Teenagers speak of a traumatic exam at school. Parents talk about the trauma of a child starting school. Young adults bemoan the trauma of dating. But the real substance of trauma is greater and deeper than these casual references would allow: Trauma is overwhelming psychological threat.

Susan Sgroi, a clinical researcher who specializes in sexual abuse cases, uses these words, saying that to be traumatized is "to come face to face with human vulnerability in the natural world and with the capacity for evil in human nature." Perhaps the most powerful simple characterizations is an event from which you never fully recover. To use more conventionally psychological terms, trauma is the simultaneous experience of extremely powerful negative feelings (overwhelming arousal) coupled with thoughts that are beyond normal ideas of human reality (overwhelming cognitions).

However we define it, trauma is and always has been a powerful force in human development. That's a sad fact of our existence on this planet, and has been since human beings emerged 200,000 years ago. Tigers, wolves, and bears mauled us. Storms, earthquakes, and fires terrified us. Other humans attacked us. And we adapted as a species.

As psychiatrist Bruce Perry has concluded from his research into the evolutionary biology underlying normal development and maturation, dealing with trauma has affected our evolution as a species. Those who found a way to adapt to trauma survived; those who did not dropped out of the gene pool. Perry notes that this

J. Garbarino, *Children and the Dark Side of Human Experience.*
© Springer Science+Business Media, LLC 2008

process of adaptation meant different things for adults than it did for children (and to some degree for adult males versus adult females). For example, adults—particularly males—who fought or fled were likely to survive. Children (and to a lesser degree women, particularly lactating women caring for children) rarely had either option. If they fought they would be summarily killed by the stronger (male) enemy adults. If they fled, they would die alone without the necessary support of friendly adults.

Thus, children (and to some degree women) were more likely to survive attack if they froze and emotionally disconnected. In this state they were less likely to be killed by an attacking enemy and more likely to survive, either by being taken into the enemy's society and raised by them as one of their own, or by waiting until their own group could reclaim them. Thus, as Perry sees it, on evolutionary grounds today's children (and to some degree women) are less likely to experience a fight-or-flight response to traumatic situations, and more likely to experience "emotional dissociation and freezing" because they are "wired" that way.

How adult human beings experience trauma has a lot to do with the way we view the world and our place in it, and how we serve as role models for the next generation (generally and even specifically when we lead families as parents or classrooms as professional teachers). People experience the effects of trauma differently, and trauma produces more severe effects in some people than others. It seems clear that some people approach traumatic events with what has been called "hardiness." For example, research by psychologist George Bonanno finds that soldiers who are rated high on hardiness before they go off to war are less likely to suffer symptoms of trauma or serious depression when they go through combat.

Others resist the effects of traumatic experiences by developing unrealistically positive views of themselves, repressing memories of the events to avoid confronting them, and practicing positive emotions to displace sadness, grief, and anger. In moderation all of these may contribute to successful coping. But if all this is simply a short-term strategy to cover over unresolved disturbing thoughts and feelings it probably will not succeed in the long run. This is not hardiness so much as it is short-sighted denial. True hardiness seems to be the most promising avenue for dealing with the horrors of the world, because it is more than simply refusing to confront traumatic experiences through self-delusion or repression, it is a matter of coping with adversity through positive strength.

What are the elements of this true hardiness? One is commitment rather than alienation. Those who do not withdraw socially and philosophically show greater resistance to the effects of experiencing traumatic events. In the face of the traumatic events one teenager may say, "No matter what happens I still believe there is goodness in the world," whereas a second responds with, "I think all you can do is get as far away as you can and just forget about it."

A second component of true hardiness is feeling in control rather than feeling powerless. It is understandable that if kids feel totally out of control they are more likely to succumb to the psychological and philosophical effects of traumatic events. One child responds, "There are things I can do to stay safe," whereas another says, "I am completely at the mercy of those who are trying to hurt me; there's nothing

I can do about it." A third element of hardiness is seeing the world in terms of challenge rather than threat. One kid says, "We can find ways to make things more peaceful and I can be a part of those efforts," whereas another says, "All I feel is fear; fear that it will happen again and there is nothing I can do about it."

Although hardiness is essential, we must be careful not to assume that kids who are coping well with trauma in their day-to-day activities (functional resilience) are necessarily at peace inside (existential resilience). I have known traumatized people who are very competent and successful on the outside but who are tormented on the inside.

Related to this point is the fact that it is not enough to look at the effects of trauma in the short run. Some people maintain functional resilience for long periods—even for decades—while falling prey to trauma-induced existential despair later. A study of Dutch resistance fighters who were involved in the struggle against the occupying Nazi forces during World War II revealed that eventually *all* of them showed some effects of their traumatic experiences, although in some cases it was not until decades later.

One of the forces at work in living with trauma is the fact that memories of the emotions of trauma do not decay; they remain fresh. My mother was a child during the bombing of London during World War II, more than half a century ago, and yet each time a new war starts she is forced to relive her childhood fear. I remember speaking with her on the phone at the start of the 1991 Gulf War, when the night-time CNN coverage of the US-led attacks on Baghdad brought the sights and sounds of bombing home via the TV set. I held the phone and listened to her sobbing as she recalled her own fear and terror.

Once you have the feeling of danger, it takes very little new threat to sustain it. In fact, it only requires an occasional re-supply of threat to keep fear alive. Psychologists who study learning find that patterns of behavior and feeling last longest when they get "intermittent" reinforcement; that is, when the reinforcement only comes infrequently rather than being constant. This is why gambling is such an easy pattern to learn and a hard one to break. You rarely win, but when you do it is enough to keep you coming back over and over again; and it is why children's fears are hard to stop once they take hold.

Trauma changes you forever. The discussion of the timing and form of trauma's effects, immediate versus long-term, and through social behavior versus internal feelings and attitudes, alerts us to the complex challenges we face in understanding how to deal with traumatic events. The psychological boundaries children bring to trauma are less well developed; thus, they are more vulnerable and trauma can more readily impinge directly on day-to-day emotional well-being. Perhaps equally important, when our psychological and philosophical resources are less well developed, it is likely that what happens really happens—in the sense captured by the characterization of trauma as "an event from which you never fully recover."

Whether or not being in a horrible situation actually registers is to some degree a matter of age (and thus stage of development). When I was in Kuwait for UNICEF at the end of the Gulf War in 1991, I witnessed an example of this first-hand. A Kuwaiti mother described how she had escaped from Kuwait one night early in the months of the Iraqi occupation of her country. She told her two daughters that they were going to play "the escape game." "In this game," she told the girls, "you have to be very quiet and stay close to me in the darkness while we walk to our friend's car." Her 5-year-old daughter accepted this as a game and nothing more, and as a result was calm during the whole ordeal. Her 10-year-old daughter, on the other hand, realized that the "game" was really a dangerous escape act and knew that if they were caught the consequences would be terrible. She was terrified until they reached safety in Saudi Arabia, and even then had bad dreams about the experience for weeks following it.

This same theme was developed in the 1997 academy award–winning film "Life Is Beautiful," in which an Italian Jewish father (Guido) shields his young son (Joshua) from the horrors of being interned in a concentration camp by persuading him it is all actually a game. It's excruciating and inspiring to watch the lengths to which Guido goes to protect his son. So long as children can live within the cocoon of these protective adult-created worlds they can and do feel safe.

When the cocoon bursts, however, young children are especially vulnerable to trauma. This, I think, is evident in the results of a general review of the topic conducted by psychiatrist Kenneth Fletcher. He reports that 27% of teenagers, 33% of middle schoolers, and 39% of younger children exhibit serious psychological symptoms when they actually encounter traumatic events. Although lower than the rate for young children, the 27% figure for teenagers is still quite significant.

Psychologists Davidson and Smith found that when exposed to comparable potentially traumatic events, 56% of children 10 or younger experienced these same symptoms compared with 18% of those 11 and older. A study conducted on the effects of a flash flood that demolished an entire town in West Virginia in 1972 (the Buffalo Creek disaster), reported that the group most vulnerable were children between the ages of 6 and 11. This is just what you would expect in the real world in which parents try to protect children from trauma. In that world, younger children are more willing and able to be protected, teenagers are more able to protect themselves, and children between these two groups are in the most vulnerable position of all, aware but relatively defenseless.

When it is tied to politics, trauma is inextricably linked to terrorism. Indeed, terrorism is all about traumatizing the enemy. In the 1979 movie "Apocalypse Now," a renegade American Special Forces officer fighting in the Vietnam War—Colonel Walter Kurtz (played by Marlon Brando)—speaks with gruesome admiration for his enemy's understanding of this.

He describes an incident in which he and his troops entered a village to inoculate the children against childhood diseases as a way of winning over the minds and hearts of the people in an area being contested by the enemy (the Viet Cong), only to return a week later to discover that the enemy had cut off the arm of each child so inoculated as a way to terrorize the population. "Pure terror," he calls it, the recognition that the enemy was willing to do anything to advance their cause, even to the point of cutting off the arms of children whose only crime was that they had been inoculated against measles and polio.

To witness such an action would be truly traumatic; it evokes overwhelming negative arousal and overwhelming negative cognitions. Even to know about it is profoundly disturbing, because once you know about the dark side of human experience things never look the same to you. Trauma really is an event that changes you forever, because it lets you in on the dark side of the human universe.

I experienced this awareness of the dark side of human experience on a visit to Cambodia in 1988. My colleagues and I were taken to see an elementary school that had been used as a torture and execution center by the murderous Khmer Rouge regime. Preserved as a museum, it stands as a monument to trauma. Even more articulate, however, were the "killing fields." In one location that we visited, some 20,000 people had been executed and dumped into mass graves. The site had been excavated—most of the remains had been removed—but as the rain fell that day it still exposed bones. In the center of the 2-acre site was a monument, a tower of skulls arranged by age—the skulls of infants and young children at the bottom, then adolescents, then adults. Off to the right a few feet was a tree—like an oak tree—that was used to kill babies: just hold them by their feet and swing their skulls against the trunk.

Having this information in your head is what "overwhelming cognitions" is all about. To have seen and heard and smelled it happening would have constituted the "overwhelming arousal." To have both together would have been authentically traumatizing, and I agree with psychiatrist Lenore Terr, who says that authentic traumatization requires both.

What are the effects of such traumatization on children and youth? Beyond the immediate psychological effects of this kind of trauma are effects that I think of as philosophical. By philosophical, I mean the effects of trauma on the way kids understand the meaning of life. These effects include a loss of confidence in the future, a decline in seeing a purpose to living, and a reduction of belief in the institutions of the community and larger society. I have seen this often in kids living in violent situations without anticipation of solution and hope. They sometimes adopt a stance of "terminal thinking," as when you ask a 15 year old what he expects to be when he is 30 and he answers, "dead."

I have witnessed all these consequences of trauma in my work as an expert witness in murder trials: Most of the criminals I sit and talk with are best understood as untreated traumatized children inhabiting adolescent or adult bodies.

Trauma comes in many forms, but at its core are what I think of as Three Dark Secrets. The first secret is that despite the comforting belief that we are physically strong and durable, the fact of the matter is that the human body can easily be maimed or destroyed by acts of physical violence. Images of graphic violence demonstrate the reality of this proposition.

I call this Snowden's Secret, after a character in Joseph Heller's 1961 novel, *Catch-22*, who is grievously wounded during a World War II mission on an American military aircraft. Hit by antiaircraft fire, airman Snowden appears have suffered only a minor injury when first approached by fellow crewman Yossarian. But when Snowden complains of feeling cold, Yossarian opens the young man's flak jacket, at which point Snowden's insides spill out onto the floor. This reveals Snowden's secret, that the human body, which appears so strong and durable, is actually just a fragile bag filled with gooey stuff and lumps, suspended on a brittle skeleton that is no match for steel. Otherwise sheltered individuals can learn this secret from their visual exposure to terrorist attacks, and it is one of the principal sources of trauma for most of us.

I remember vividly watching TV in the first hours of the attack on 9/11 and watching a young man in suit and tie recall to the interviewer that he had watched someone jump from the 100th floor of the World Trade Center tower and fall to his death, actually seeing this victim hit the pavement. With a stunned look and a pathetic voice the witness said, "I will never be the same after this." He's right.

The second secret is that the social fabric is as vulnerable as the physical body; that despite all their power and authority, our parents and leaders cannot necessarily keep us safe when an enemy wishes us harm. This is most evident with respect to children and their relationships with parents, teachers, and other adults, but it has currency for adults as well.

I call this Dantrell's Secret, in commemoration of a little boy in Chicago who, in 1992, was walked to school by his mother. When they arrived, teachers stood on the steps of the school and a police car was positioned at the street corner. Nonetheless, as 7-year-old Dantrell Davis walked the 75 feet from his mother to his teacher he was shot in the head and killed by a sniper in a gang-related shooting. Learning this secret can turn otherwise good citizens away from the structures of ordinary community authority to fend for themselves out of a sense of self-defensive adaptation, knowing now that your leaders cannot protect you, that the social fabric of community power and authority is as fragile as the human body.

It is a message that many American children learned with particular poignancy on September 11, 2001, as they watched the planes crash into the World Trade Center towers, over and over again, and again as they saw adults watch helplessly as the buildings collapsed minutes later. It is a secret that millions of children the world over have learned from being exposed to political violence in all its forms.

The third is Milgram's Secret, the knowledge that anything is possible when it comes to violence; there are no limits to human savagery. Stanley Milgram was a Yale University psychologist who conducted what was certainly among the most controversial experiments ever performed by an American social scientist. He organized a study in which volunteers for an experiment on "memory" were positioned in front of a control board designed to allow them as "teacher" to administer electric shocks to an unseen "learner." The question underlying the study was: Would the "teachers" administer what they knew were painful electric shocks to the "learners" if they were told it was their duty to do so?

Before conducting the experiment Milgram surveyed people as to what they thought would happen in his experiment. Most people said that they thought "normal" people would refuse to inflict such torture and that only a few "crazy" sadists would do so. The results of the study were that, although many participants were uncomfortable doing so, 65% of the "teachers" administered the torture—sometimes cursing the "learners" as they did so. This is Milgram's Secret, that comforting assumptions about what is and is not possible all disintegrate in the face of the human capacity to commit violence "for a good purpose."

Milgram's Secret is coming to grips with the fact that any form of violence that can be imagined can be committed so long as the perpetrator believes he is justified in doing so. How many ways are there to kill and maim a human being? The news confronts children with the varieties of death and dying. Is there any form of mutilation that is out of bounds and beyond human possibility? Survivors of Nazi death camps, the Pol Pot Khmer Rouge terror in Cambodia, and abusive families know that the answer is no. Children and youth who watch TV know it too. Anything is possible. It will take a long time to help children recover from all the traumatic images that flood over them.

True believers will fly planes into buildings at the cost of their own and thousands of other lives. True believers will strap explosives on their bodies, walk into a school full of children, and detonate the explosives. True believers will spread lethal chemical, biological, and radioactive toxins in the food and water of a community. Whatever can be imagined can be done. Learning this secret can drive anyone, but particularly those who are psychologically or philosophically vulnerable, to emotional shut down or hedonistic self-destruction.

How do human beings learn these three dark secrets? In my experience, some learn them the old-fashioned way, by experiencing them first-hand as the result of abuse, natural disaster, suffering a horrible accident, witnessing a violent crime, or living in a war zone. I've met all these people. A child in Omaha said of his abusive mother, "She could kill me," and he's right. A girl in Nicaragua lived through an earthquake and said, "The ground started to move and the buildings fell down and I watched my mother die." A New York teenager grew sad and quiet and talked of dropping out of school after he recklessly drove the family car into a telephone pole and caused the death of his three passengers, parts of whose bodies ended up on his clothing because they were not wearing seat belts and so were dismembered upon impact.

A young girl in Chicago played dead and watched as her mother was raped and killed by an intruder, and she did not speak for 4 weeks. A little boy in Croatia told the story of how enemy soldiers came to his village and took his brother and father, and then, when asked to draw a picture of "life now" drew the body of a boy floating face down in the ocean. Two brothers in Kuwait told of how they found an unexploded grenade after the Iraqi soldiers retreated in 1991, and they began to toss it around like a ball with their 10-year-old cousin until it exploded and killed him and cost one of the boys the sight in his left eye.

The commonly used term for the package of psychological symptoms that occur after traumatic experiences is posttraumatic stress disorder (PTSD). This term arose from the demands of Vietnam War veterans for official psychiatric recognition of what they were experiencing. The vets wanted the diagnosis to be called catastrophic stress disorder, but for a variety of technical reasons, psychiatrists preferred posttraumatic stress disorder. Professionals working with other groups that had experienced horrific events (rape victims, sexual abuse victims, natural disaster victims) saw the utility of this term, and the label has stuck in both professional circles and the public mind.

Recently, there has been criticism of both the intellectual and practical value of the diagnosis, however. For example, psychotherapist Bonnie Burstow argues that PTSD is not a valid or useful concept, and that the criteria for the diagnosis are at best confused and at worst destructive. For one thing, the "symptoms" included in the diagnosis may actually be adaptive efforts to cope with horror. As Burstow writes, "What is not pleasant becomes a symptom and, as such, is pathologized" (p. 432). For example, recurrent dreams may be a way of working through the meaning of experiences. The same goes for avoiding situations that remind you of the trauma: This can be adaptive (at least at first, and from time to time) to prevent being overwhelmed.

A second problem with the PTSD diagnosis is that it strips away the potential meaning that an individual may derive from encounters with horror. As Burstow puts it:

> People who are not traumatized maintain the illusion of safety moment to moment by editing out such facets as the pervasiveness of war, the subjugation of women and children, everyday racist violence, religious intolerance, the frequency and unpredictability of natural disasters, the ever-present threat of sickness and death and so on. People who have been badly traumatized are less likely to edit out these very real dimensions of reality. Once traumatized, they are not longer shielded from reality by a cloak of invulnerability. (p. 435)

What's more, the PTSD diagnosis seems to fly in the face of accumulating evidence from psychological research on what is more and more coming to be called "positive psychology." Traumatic events can be the impetus for growth and development, not just psychopathology. Beyond resilience—bouncing back to normal after experiencing a traumatic event—lies what some psychologists have called "adversarial growth." It's a happy event that research is demonstrating the reality of growth in response to trauma. I say "happy" for two reasons. First, the lives of many children are filled with trauma, and thus any good news about this inevitability is encouraging and sustaining. Second, it provides systematic validation for a great deal of folk wisdom—"that which does not kill me strengthens me," and "kites rise against, not with, the wind." Although not inviting trauma proactively, these responses do offer some hope of making good developmental use of trauma if it cannot be avoided.

Protecting children from trauma is one of the principal human rights challenges we face. It has always been so. But now in the twenty-first century we face this challenge in a new technological context, in which vicarious traumatization becomes possible as media images are crafted and communicated with historically unprecedented power. The experience of terrorism for children of the "age of mass media" illustrates this issue.

Case Study: 9/11 and the Problem of Vicarious Trauma

Fortunately, relatively few American kids have been subjected to the kinds of traumatic lessons that afflict children growing up in war zones, refugee camp, and violent neighborhoods, but the events of 9/11 served this nasty purpose for large numbers of the current generation of children and youth. Here's Laura's moving account of how she learned the three dark secrets of trauma. Now a 21-year-old college student, on September 11, 2001, she was a high school student in New York City, and offers a vivid account of what "overwhelming arousal" and "overwhelming cognition" mean to a sensitive soul. Every detail of her account is worth hearing because it captures the essence of trauma and resilience:

> My high school (Stuyvesant) was a couple of blocks from the World Trade Center. I was in math class when we heard the crash of the first plane into the building. It sounded like a missile, and we looked outside and saw the billowing smoke. Our principal told us it was an accident, but we put the TV on in our classroom and saw another plane hit the other tower—an even weirder experience because we heard it outside our windows simultaneously. It felt so surreal; I felt like I couldn't breathe. I knew my mom had gone shopping there that morning. Other kids were on their cell phones, crying, trying to reach parents that worked there. We were still told to go to our next class and I was then on the 10th floor when the first tower collapsed. Our whole building shook and the lights flickered and students were crying, under desks hiding, screaming. We thought we'd been hit, but then my teacher told us a tower had collapsed and I somehow felt relieved. I was crying then, as we were told to go to homeroom. I looked outside and there was smoke everywhere. One side of my school was covered in a sheet of dust. Papers were flying everywhere and below, on the West Side Highway, was a mass exodus of people in work clothes, crying, covered in soot, stiletto high-heeled shoes lying on the side of the road, moving uptown. We were told to do the same—evacuate. I found my best friend and as we walked outside. I was hysterical—all those people dead for no good reason. The second tower had collapsed and as we walked uptown to my dad's office I turned back and just saw two huge columns of smoke where the towers had once stood. It was like a movie, all these people walking, nothing but dust behind us, so surreal. I knew things would never be the same. I couldn't sleep for many nights. I would close my eyes and remember the people jumping out the windows in the Trade Center—at the time I had noticed them, but I didn't think those "colors" were people that were standing on the ledges. Our school was closed for almost a month and used as a rest center for the fireman. For a couple of weeks we attended half-day sessions at another high school. No one questioned it; there was this new understanding and tightness among my classmates. When we returned to lower Manhattan it was a war zone. I remember the smell, the lights at night, the Army tanks, the emptiness and sadness, the construction and sheer desolation. I don't know how we all got back on track, how we applied for college, but we did. Things slowly got better, and today when I go down there it's a tourist attraction. It's almost like nothing happened. Businesses are booming once more, but I remember 9/11 and what came after, my senior year when I took the subway and was warned of bio-terrorism and anthrax and new attacks. I'm not scared anymore, but I won't forget when I was.

Laura had a lot going for her in confronting the horror and its aftermath. She has many elements of resilience and robustness. She is smart. She has strong family support and access to social, economic, and educational assets and resources. Being so close to the site of the attacks, her school was enrolled in a mental health program aimed at providing psychological first aid to the students and faculty. She is emotionally healthy. She did not lose a family member or close friend in the disaster. She was an adolescent when the trauma came upon her. And, very importantly, her life before and after 9/11 was free of horror. But she and other kids like her face some unprecedented issues related to trauma (as well as benefiting from historically new mental health interventions designed to deal with its effects).

Historically, the origins of trauma have generally been limited to first-hand encounters with horror, such as what Laura experienced on 9/11; but things have changed. The media technologies that emerged in the twentieth century added a new, unprecedented dimension to the psychology of terror by opening us all to trauma induced by the vicarious experience of horror in full-spectrum imagery and sounds. This makes the experience of kids in "real" war zones all the more important to understand, since their reality may more and more become our reality.

One of the important elements of living in the current age of terror is the growing recognition that modern mass media permit the conveying of traumatic experiences beyond those who are in-person witnesses, to the mass audience who are exposed to vivid visual and auditory representations of horror via videotaped records.

This was observed in post-occupation Kuwait in the early 1990s, when videotapes of Iraqi atrocities were sufficient to elicit traumatic responses in children (who identified with the victims as their countrymen, as do American children who are exposed to atrocities committed against other Americans). The same was true of video reports of the space shuttle disaster in 1986. Children who saw it were traumatized by it. Children were traumatized on an even greater scale by their media-centered experience of 9/11. They must have at the back of their minds, the question, "Will things ever be back to normal?"

The possibility—indeed the probability—of terrorist attacks has become part of the new normal. Indeed, the very "normal" to which kids refer is itself part of the problem faced by us all today. Televised images of threat and violence play a central role in modern TV and movies. In her study of children, psychologist Joanne Cantor's research demonstrates that the imagery of the movies "Jaws" and "Halloween" elicited long-lasting traumatic responses: 25% reported a fright reaction that lasted at least a year, and more than 20% reported "subsequent mental preoccupation with the frightening aspects of the stimulus."

Studies among adults report that the more TV we watch, the more suspicious and fearful we become about the social environment around us. This is an important element of the socially toxic environment in which children grow up today, in the United States and many other places in the world. Why? Because psychological connection to the immediate victims of terrorist horror is capable of transmitting trauma second-hand, and the sensory power of the mass media can make the connection for kids on a scale and with an intensity not previously available.

The stories told by kids I have listened to resonate with a study reporting that personal acquaintance with disaster victims is the most potent influence on whether or not we will exhibit stress reactions in response to a catastrophe (in the case of that study, a terrible bus accident). Thus, even though many of us know that we were geographically distanced from the World Trade Center and the Pentagon in 2001, we felt psychologically connected as Americans. One study found effects of 9/11 on the heart functioning of kids living hundreds of miles away from New York City.

Trauma is the experience of horror. Second-hand victimization via exposure to visual and auditory images of people with whom one has a psychological connection provides a mechanism for explaining indirect trauma. If movies about sharks and costumed mass murderers could resonate with traumatic impact on the youth who saw them, imagine the long-term effects of the movie "two planes hit the World Trade Center" and "bombs explode in subway" that have already premiered in the news world of the mass media. And contemplate the effects of the likely sequels, "atomic device detonated in Los Angeles," "biological toxin released in Detroit's water system," and "chemical agent poisons air in Atlanta." Understanding the meaning and means of trauma is the first step.

The second step in understanding how trauma reverberates through the culture of kids in extreme situations comes when we recognize the difference between single (acute) incidents of trauma and repeated (chronic) patterns of trauma. A single incident of trauma such as the attack of 9/11 or the experience of Hurricane Katrina is a big psychological challenge for children and teenagers. In the short run it can stimulate a range of psychological symptoms, including emotional numbing, hypervigilance, an exaggerated startle response and other problems with arousal responses, anxiety, detachment from others, disrupted play, nightmares and other sleep disturbances, and depression. All this can result from one bad day—whether witnessing a shooting, surviving a tornado, or being sexually assaulted. One study of youth living near the site of the World Trade Centers in New York City reported that 70% showed these symptoms in the immediate aftermath of the 9/11 attack. But chronic immersion of kids in traumatic imagery is increasingly common, and it is a measure of social toxicity, the topic of the next chapter.

Chapter 3
The Right to a Healthy Social Environment: Protecting Children from Social Toxicity

To live in fear and falsehood is worse than death.

—Zoroastrian text

Some kids are smarter than others. Some are better looking than others. Some are kinder and more sensitive than others. Some are more talented than others. Some are more confident than others. But all these differences pale in comparison with what kids share, and kids don't change much at their core over the years. They want to be valued and accepted. They want to be safe. They want to learn and explore. They want to play and have fun. They need to find meaning in their lives and make a spiritual connection.

It's not these core themes and concerns that change. Rather, it is the cultural, psychological, and social messages and tools they have available to them as they go about the universal business of growing up. The nature of these messages and tools does have an effect on that process of growing up, however. Some ennoble; others degrade. Some promote social order; others promote chaos. Some are good; some are bad. Some result in young adults who want to serve humanity and carve out a spiritually meaningful life for themselves, like the kids I read about who raised money in their school to help Hurricane Katrina victims a thousand miles away. Others result in teenagers like the ones I watched on a "reality" program on TV who to a person said their goal in life was "to be rich and famous."

When the social environment spreads fear and falsehood it becomes poisonous to the development of children and youth, much as when the physical environment is poisoned and misused it can undermine their physical well-being. This is particularly true for kids who are especially vulnerable to developmental harm because of their difficult temperament or mental health problems.

Social toxicity refers to the extent to which the social environment of children and youth is poisonous, in the sense that it contains serious threats to the development of identity, competence, moral reasoning, trust, hope, and the other features of personality and ideology that make for success in school, family, work, and the community. Like physical toxicity, it can be fatal—in the forms of suicide, homicide, drug-related and other life style-related preventable deaths. But mostly it results in diminished "humanity" in the lives of children and youth by virtue of leading them to live in a state of degradation, whether they know it or not.

J. Garbarino, *Children and the Dark Side of Human Experience.*
© Springer Science+Business Media, LLC 2008

What are the social and cultural poisons that are psychologically equivalent to lead and smoke in the air, PCBs in the water, and pesticides in the food chain? We can see social toxicity in the values, practices, and institutions that breed feelings of fear about the world, arrogance and entitlement feelings of rejection by adults inside and outside the family, exposure to traumatic images and experiences, absence of adult supervision, and inadequate exposure to positive adult role models. These feelings and experiences arise from being embedded in a shallow materialist culture, surrounded with negative and degrading media messages, and deprived of relationships with sources of character in the school, neighborhood, and larger community.

For example, research on the impact of televised violence indicates that its effect on increasing aggressive behavior by child viewers is equivalent to the effect of smoking on lung cancer—namely that it accounts for about 10–15% of the variation. In this sense, violent TV is a social toxin. By the same token, all the various "-isms"—for example, racism and sexism—that diminish the worth of targeted groups are toxins in the sense that they are linked to negative developmental outcomes.

The bias against homosexuals has a similarly negative effect. Although the term homophobia is widely accepted, it may not be the most useful way to approach this issue, as it allows offending bigots to say, "I don't fear homosexuals, I just don't like them and think they are unnatural or deviant." There is no widely accepted alternative: Terms such as homonegativity and heterosexualism are offered but not widely used in public.

Although it took decades of advocacy, the professional psychological community has finally acknowledged that there is no scientific foundation for whatever we may call the bias against homosexuals. For example, in 1973 the American Psychiatric Association's Board of Trustees declared that "homosexuality per se implies no impairment in judgment, stability, reliability, or general social or vocational capabilities," and came out squarely against public and private discrimination against gays and lesbians.

This has not ended homophobic actions, of course. A study of high school students published in 1998 found that in comparison with heterosexual kids, gay, lesbian, and bisexual youth were five times more likely to miss school because they felt unsafe, four times more likely to be threatened with a weapon at school, twice as likely to have their property damaged at school, and three times more likely to require medical treatment after a fight at school, despite the fact that they were four times *less* likely to be involved in fighting at school.

The social toxin of homophobia can be fatal, as I learned in the death of a college friend. I started college at St. Lawrence University, a small liberal arts college in northern New York State in 1964, and, like many male college freshman of that era, soon became part of a group of guys that regularly played touch football in the fall and spring, attended hockey games in the winter, and went out to the movies and the bars most weekends for the next 4 years. There was nothing remarkable about our little group of 10 regular guys, except perhaps that our grade point average was a good bit above the norms for our cohort of students and few of us ended up joining a fraternity (which made us a minority on campus at the time).

After graduation I lost touch with most of them, except my best friend in the group, Dan, who moved first to Germany and then to Colorado, while I stayed in the East. About 10 years after we graduated I spoke to Dan on the phone in one of our irregular catching-up sessions. He told me he had tracked down one of the members of our group—I will call him "Dave". Not having an up-to-date address for him, Dan had called Dave's old home phone number and reached his mother. After some awkward preliminaries she told Dan that Dave was dead. He had committed suicide 2 years earlier. Dan was devastated—as was I when I heard the news.

Why had this smart and very "normal" young man taken his own life? His mother explained to Dan that Dave had left a note saying he was gay and that the shame and fear of being exposed were too much for him. So he ended his life before it had hardly begun. I was shocked, both because of Dave's death and by the realization that he had not trusted us, his friends, with his secret. Looking back on it more than 40 years later I can understand his reluctance.

In the mid-1960s the bias against gay boys and men was much more uniform and unthinkingly righteous than it is today among college students. I can't honestly say how the other guys in our group would have responded to discovering his secret. I like to think that I would have been accepting. I like to think that the others would have followed suit. I like to think that, but when I recall the way we all joked about the guys in our dorm who we suspected were gay because of their effeminate mannerisms I am not so sure. Certainly Dave didn't think he could take the risk.

Of course, knowing what we know now—that about 10% of human beings are homosexual in their orientation—it should not be surprising that among 10 young men one would be gay. This new awareness today does not mean that boys and young men are automatically and universally free to be who they are, of course. A study my colleagues and I conducted with college students in the late 1990s revealed that although 10% of both the males and females said that they realized they were gay or lesbian while they were in high school, only a minority had come out to their parents (only 10% of the girls and 40% of the boys).

As reported earlier, it was not until 1973 that the American Psychiatric Association's Board of Trustees declared that "homosexuality per se" is not pathological, and came out squarely against public and private discrimination against gays and lesbians. Things have changed for the better on this fundamental issue of human rights, the right to be who you are, albeit too late for my friend Dave. Now many more people are comfortable with the idea of homosexuality and in relationship with real live homosexuals, and many more gay and lesbian individuals feel safe enough to come out. A cursory tour through prime time TV and mainstream movies makes that clear.

But rejection and hatred directed at gays and lesbians is one of the few forms of negative bias that can still be expressed openly in America by politicians, religious leaders, and other public figures. After all, even as late as 1998 the American Psychiatric Association's Board of Trustees thought it necessary to issue a statement saying it opposes any psychiatric treatment based upon the assumption that homosexuality per se is a mental disorder of the a priori assumption that a patient should want to or try to change his or her sexual orientation. Also, it is still true that openly homosexual individuals are barred from serving in the U.S. military—and they continue to be discharged once their "secret" is officially acknowledged. My friend Dave died from the social toxicity of homophobia, and until it is exorcised from our culture kids who are gay or lesbian will not be safe.

Homophobia, racism, sexism: All these dimensions of social toxicity are important, but superseding and infusing them all is spiritual emptiness, the loss of a sense of living in a positive meaningful universe beyond the material experience of day-to-day life. When there is no meaning beyond the material there is no life beyond going to the shopping mall. I heard this once in its most terrible form when a 19 year old who had just been sentenced to life in prison (for killing a police officer) said he was going to kill himself. "Why?" I asked. "Because I am never going to the mall again," he replied. Indeed, if kids live only for their commercial lives, there really is no life left when denied access to the shopping mall that gives their lives material meaning.

Just as some children are more vulnerable than others to physical poisons in the ground and air, some children are more vulnerable to social toxicity. Emotionally troubled and temperamentally vulnerable children living in a socially toxic environment are like psychological asthmatics living in an atmospherically polluted city. It seems young children are most vulnerable to aspects of life that threaten the availability and quality of care by parents and other caregivers; whereas adolescents are most vulnerable to toxic influences in the broader culture and community, such as pornography on the Internet and violent video games in the mall.

Adolescence is mostly and usually the crystallization of childhood experience, so the youth most at risk are those who develop psychological vulnerabilities in childhood and then face social deprivation and trauma in adolescence. This is why research reveals that in some (positive) neighborhoods, only 15% of 9-year-old children who have developed a chronic pattern of aggression, bad behavior, acting out, and violating the rights of others—kids who might be diagnosed with conduct disorder—become serious violent delinquents; in other (negative) neighborhoods the figure is 60%!

At-risk and marginalized youth act as social weathervanes in the sense that they indicate the direction of social change in their societies. The particular cultural and social pathologies present in a society generally are most evident in the lives of these youth. For example, when the old Soviet system in Eastern Europe collapsed, adolescent drug abuse became epidemic. The epidemic in Thailand and the Philippines is child prostitution. When the drug economy overwhelmed the justice system, murderous youth violence became epidemic in Colombia.

In each case, psychologically vulnerable youth were most affected. They are the youth who already have accumulated the most developmental risk factors: youth who enter adolescence with a history of malfunctioning families, youth with unstable and reactive temperaments, and youth with emotional disabilities.

The moral compass of character grounded in spiritual realization is the tool kids need to help them through the ethical complexities of the lives they live in real life. Character education is all about setting out the core values that kids and adults will strive to live by, the standards they will set for themselves as decent people, knowing full well they don't always measure up. None of us does.

Character takes us toward evaluating our imperfect attempts to be good in light of how well our behavior conforms to the core values of trustworthiness, respect, responsibility, fairness, caring, and citizenship. The real test for anyone is to answer this question, "If you had the choice of a million dollars or a solid character, which would you choose?" That is the real question, not, "Are you a morally perfect person?" We are not perfect, but we can seek to live with character.

One school I visited had the following slogan on the cafeteria wall: "Character is what you do when no one is looking." Point well taken, but probably more important still is the realization that "Character is what you do when your peers are looking," for peers are the vehicle for enforcing the soulless culture of contemporary shallow materialism. This was evident when a student at that same high school told me the real, unspoken slogan of his school was, "The strong do what they will; the weak endure what they must."

Amidst all the confusion and temptations and blind alleys of modern life, we can always gain clarity by asking, "Does this contribute to my character development?" If it doesn't, we must go back to the drawing board. Years ago a colleague of mine had a bumper sticker on his office door that read, "You can change the world ... but unless you know what you are doing, please don't."

It's a profound message for each of us. What you do does make a difference; but that does not guarantee that the difference will be one you will embrace once you see it, and its ramifications. What can we do? We can make the investment of time and energy necessary to understand more fully what we are facing, what the stakes are, and what the choices are in responding to kids in extreme situations at home and abroad.

In this life-and-death struggle against the shallow nastiness of pop culture, all life-affirming meaning for our children's character is an ally. Soul searching reveals this truth as one that applies to all children in every setting. All the physical and psychological issues of child development in extreme situations must be solved, but ultimately the fundamental issue is the one of character informed by spirituality. Like Dorothy in the Wizard of Oz, I have learned that the most important lessons of life are to be learned right in your own back yard.

Despite all the toxicity in American culture, I see a lot that is good. When I was in Kuwait in 1991 on behalf of UNICEF days after its liberation from Iraqi occupation, I was proud to be an American, as I saw how our warriors comported themselves. One group of soldiers used their few precious hours of down time to clean up a residential facility for retarded kids that had been abandoned by the staff, and was filthy and unsanitary. I witnessed a scene in which American soldiers intervened to protect some Palestinians (who were thought to have collaborated with the Iraqi occupation) from assault by a Kuwaiti military unit. Closer to home, I have witnessed innumerable examples of American generosity, some private, some public. Certainly the outpouring of volunteers and contributions in the wake of the South Asia tsunami and Hurricane Katrina exemplified what is best in America.

But the nature of my work has also exposed me to some of the dark side of America, and its moral and political limitations. I traveled to New Orleans in 2006, a year after the Katrina Hurricane hit, and I saw reconstruction mired in racism, the interests of the affluent class trumping the needs of the poor, and politics as usual. Two years later there are still reports that emergency aid has been diverted and wasted, to the detriment of meeting the basic needs of many residents of the city.

I have been to Cambodia and seen how American arrogance during the Vietnam War in the 1960s and 1970s all but guaranteed the success of Pol Pot's Khmer Rouge in taking over the country, and thus setting in motion the years of insane slaughter that followed. I have been to Nicaragua and seen the toll taken on lives and spirits by American support for the Contras' war against the Sandinistas during the 1980s. I have been to the Middle East repeatedly and seen how decades of American pro-Israeli bias and unwillingness to recognize the legitimate national aspirations of the Palestinians allowed that conflict to fester and continue to the ugly point it has reached today.

Perhaps most to the point, among all the nearly 150 nations of the world the United States stands nearly alone (one of only two U.N. members that have not ratified the U.N. Convention on the Rights of the Child—the other being Somalia, which can at least offer the defense that it does not have a functioning central government empowered to enact ratification). Two toxic forces have blocked ratification. The first is the fundamentalist impulse in American culture that fears and rejects human rights initiatives in general as a threat to the power of the entrenched interests of homophobic, patriarchal, punishment-oriented "traditional values."

The second is the power of those who believe we are above and beyond the rest of the world ("We're number one!"), and therefore entitled to our exceptional status. Americans have a special difficulty in dealing with this issue. One of our problems is what historians have called our "historical exceptionalism." What they mean by this term is that we tend to view our history as unique, and to reject the idea that we are like everyone else, as a people and as a country. It is a rare politician who can refrain from saying, "This is the greatest nation on Earth." Many would go so far as to say this is the greatest nation that has ever existed, unique among all countries.

The theme of exceptionalism reverberates down through the decades of American history. Historian Amy Kaplan sees it at work in the language used to described the events and sequelae of the 9/11 attacks. For example, the area around the destroyed World Trade Centers is called "Ground Zero." As Kaplan points out, the term was coined to describe the atomic attacks on Hiroshima and Nagasaki in August 1945, yet we never hear these catastrophes cited as cataclysmic catastrophes in any way analogous to the events of 9/11. Rather, the most common analogy offered to and by the public is the December 7, 1942 attack on Pearl Harbor.

Kaplan writes that on the face of it, this is odd because "the experience of a sudden, horrific attack on civilians in an urban center seems in fact, much more like the events of September 11 than the Japanese attack on a U.S. naval base" (pp. 83–84). She continues, "The term Ground Zero both evokes and eclipses the prior historical reference, using it as a yardstick of terror—to claim that this was just like the horrific experience of a nuclear bomb—while at the same time consigning the prior reference to historical amnesia" (p. 84). So why refer to Pearl Harbor but not Hiroshima-Nagasaki?

There are at least two major differences between Pearl Harbor and Hiroshima-Nagasaki. First, from the American perspective the former was unjust and the latter was just, because we were not in a formal state of war with Japan in 1941 and we were in 1945. What about September 11, 2001? The official claim is that we were the innocent victims of unprovoked assault by the forces of evil. Certainly the individuals working in the World Trade Centers were innocent victims by virtue of their civilian status; but anyone familiar with the dark side of American policy and interventions in the Middle East during the second half of the twentieth century—including Iraq and Iran—could be forgiven for questioning our national innocence in that region.

Noam Chomsky, among others, has made it clear that as a nation we have put our material national interests above our beloved commitment to democracy—particularly as these interests coalesce in the matter of access to petroleum. After all, we supported Saddam Hussein's regime in Iraq right up to the point where it invaded Kuwait and threatened Saudi Arabia (our oil friends and allies despite their non-democratic character and nurturing the religious fanaticism of most of the 9/11 terrorists).

Of course, to many non-Americans, the most obvious difference is that America was both the target in 1941 and the nation that did the targeting in 1945, not to mention the fact that the casualties inflicted in 1945 by American forces were much, much larger than those incurred by the United States on either December 7, 1941, or September 11, 2001. Given the historically unprecedented magnitude of the destruction wrought by the arrival of the atomic bombs in Hiroshima and Nagasaki in August 1945, that attack was no doubt as much a "surprise attack" to the Japanese civilians as the use of airliners as "suicide bombers" on 9/11 was to New Yorkers of 2001. To the best of my knowledge, no Japanese leaders received a briefing in July 1945 entitled "Uncle Sam poised to use atomic weapons for attack on Japan" (although there were those in the government who proposed offering Japan just such a warning, perhaps including a demonstration of the weapon). This stands in contrast to the fact that American officials received an intelligence briefing in the summer of 2001 highlighting al Qaeda's fascination with the prospect of using airplanes as bombs to produce spectacular casualties. We need some humility and historical perspective to balance our national sense entitlement and self-centered inflated ego.

What we do matters in our own lives, in the larger world, and for the future. It matters in our public policies, our social programs, and our sense of ourselves as moral beings. It matters to our ability to live a soulful existence, one that meets our spiritual needs. This is all the more reason for us to have the deepest, most sophisticated analysis of the issues that confront and surround us as we seek to nurture the human rights of children and youth in our society and around the world. I think we can start this process by looking backward, to the America of the 1950s.

America in the 1950s had just emerged from the Great Depression and World War II. During the Great Depression in the 1930s large numbers of American workers were unemployed because of the economic crisis, and felt despair, fear, and anger that through no fault of their own they were being impoverished. Debate continues among historians and economists about the exact causes of the Depression and the strategies and tactics used to deal with it by the national government and other public policy entities. What does seem clear is that the actions of President Franklin Roosevelt, a Democrat elected to lead the nation in 1932, played an important role in inspiring demoralized unemployed workers, who prior to his arrival on the national scene felt betrayed and abandoned by the national political leadership and business leaders who were their allies. The renowned American writer John Updike was a child during the 1930s and recalls observing his own unemployed father's desolation, and his reaction to the policies and words of President Roosevelt:

> My father had been reared a Republican, but he switched parties to vote for Roosevelt and never switched back. His memory of being abandoned by society and big business never left him and, for all his paternal kindness and humorousness, communicated itself to me, along with his preference for the political party that offered "the forgotten man" the better break. Roosevelt made such people feel less alone. The impression of recovery—the impression that a President was bending the old rules and, drawing upon his own courage and flamboyance in adversity and illness, stirring things up on behalf of the down-and-out—mattered more than any miscalculations in the moot mathematics of economics.

World War II built upon this sense of meaningfulness to create a powerful sense of confidence and solidarity. Tom Brokaw captured all this in his book, *The Greatest Generation*, and this was the launching pad for the 1950s. Despite the challenges parents of the 1950s faced with the rise of atomic war as a threat, I believe they had an easier time of it when it came to protecting children than I did as a parent in the 1980s and 1990s, and than do parents in the world of the twenty-first century. For one thing, the flow of information to children 50 years ago was under relatively tight and benign control. To be sure, this control had a down side (e.g., in its narrow portrayal of females and ethnic and racial minorities and the absence of people with other than heterosexual orientation); but on the plus side, TV was effectively censored when it came to sex and vivid violence.

There was a strong sense that "children are watching," and this meant that adults should forego the pleasure and titillation of explicit sexuality on the screen. Of course, this censorship limited the ability of TV and movies to deal with some adult subjects, but in retrospect I don't think the cost was too great. Themes of sexuality, infidelity, debilitating illness, depression, suicide, and murder could be presented, but in a manner that seems muted, dignified, and subtle by today's "let it all hang out" standards.

There was violence, but it was highly stylized and sanitized. The bad guys were only moderately nasty, and the good guys subscribed to a strict code of honorable conduct. In the TV environment of the 1950s, even the child of a negligent parent was at little risk sitting in front of the TV set, because the narrow range of available images and themes was tightly controlled by the adults who made and broadcast the programming. The same was true for movies.

The media technology of the 1950s also worked to the advantage of children. Special effects were primitive and not likely to produce the kind of visual trauma associated with contemporary images of violence, horror, and depravity. The cumbersome quality of visual recording technology—limited for the most part to film—reduced to negligible the possibility that horrific events would be made available visually to the TV and movie viewer, including the child viewer.

Today, the ubiquitous availability of video recording means that much of what is horrible to see will be made available for the seeing, and usually by children as readily as adults. Consider the horror of the attack on Pearl Harbor in 1941 versus the attack on the World Trade Center 60 years later. The former was visually witnessed by a relative handful of children; the latter was seen via videotape by virtually every child in America—over and over again, in many cases. Repeat this for every violent and traumatic image over and over again, from the big events like plane crashes to the little events like ritual beatings purveyed over local TV news as well as over You Tube and other Internet sites that cater to kids. This exposure to traumatic imagery is one important feature of the social toxicity that compounds the problem of parents and other caring adults in helping children deal with growing up in the age of terror, but it is not the only element.

As the atomic age began, the structure of benevolent adult authority was relatively intact, at least when compared to the world of twenty-first-century America. Adults were adults, and kids were kids. The social contract between children and adults was intact and in force: Children live in their world (under the direct supervision of empowered adults); adults live in theirs (mostly out of sight from the innocent eyes of children). Adults were in charge and in return took responsibility for protecting children.

This empowered adults to keep children out of the adult world and the institutions of America cooperated and conspired to maintain the useful illusion that children didn't have to worry because the grown-ups were taking care of business on their behalf. Perhaps one notable exception to this rule was in the duck-and-cover scare tactics associated with the threat of atomic war. The very exceptionality of this violation of children's sense of safety is evidence of the existence of the general rule of innocence.

But with each new year after 1950, children's visual access to scary stuff increased, whether horrific violence of war and crime, parental incapacitation, family break-up, the clay feet of political leaders, or the sweaty details of sexuality. Today's routine exposure of children to social toxicity means that today's child is already reeling from the sense of a broken social contract with the adult world before we even begin to factor in the challenges of living in the age of terror. Thus, if ever there was a time for parents to take up the mantle of responsibility it is now. Mediating the child's exposure to the dark side of human experience in today's already toxic social environment will continue to be one of the principal challenges for "good" parents in the years to come.

One of the casualties of both trauma and social toxicity in general is social trust and faith in the future. Adults who grew up confined to the images and messages of a child-sized world may have a solid world view to sustain their social trust and faith in the future, but children who are growing up in an age in which mass media can and do bring vivid trauma to children from an early age onward may not. A study of adults seeking psychiatric intervention found that among those who had suffered a traumatic event at a young age, nearly 75% replied yes, when they were asked, "Have you given up all hope of finding meaning in your life?" Among those who were adults before they experienced trauma the comparable figure was much lower—20%. Parents must display empathic parenting grounded in awareness of developmental processes when children are faced with trauma, lest they slip into a profound sense of meaninglessness.

For most of us, seeing life from a spiritual perspective necessitates a shift in our thinking. It requires that we see ourselves as spiritual beings first and foremost. This means that we acknowledge our spiritual identities and existence in addition to the physical and psychological realities of living as human organisms. This recognition includes awareness of the primacy of spiritual existence, a shift to recognizing oneself as a spiritual being first and foremost. Even for many who see themselves as religious, this recognition requires a fundamental shift from a materialist metaphysic of body first, consciousness second; to spirit first, body second.

What are the requisite elements of this shift? One is a transcendent organizing belief in a coherent spiritual existence (a Higher Power, a spiritual Source, a spiritual Creator, an all-benevolent higher spiritual being). Another is a belief in oneself as being connected in spirit to the Higher Power and to other human beings as other spiritual peers having a physical experience, and the centrality of love in this approach to the world. A third concerns the way we approach reality in our efforts to understand and improve it with compassion always. Each informs our analysis of how the search for meaning in the lives of children and youth facing issues of life and death makes an enormous difference in our understanding of human development. This is not just a matter of impersonal analysis. It is a matter of real lives shaped and defined by how well we do in guaranteeing each child's basic human right to a healthy social environment, how well we convert social toxicity to a socially healthy state in which all the "-isms" and other cultural poisons that affect kids are replaced with nurturing acceptance.

Case Study: The Deadly Social Toxins of Fear and Brutality in American Culture

In July 2007, I saw the Michael Moore documentary "Sicko." It's a poignant and witty look at the bizarre fact that in the United States—one of the wealthiest countries in the world—nearly 50 million Americans have no health care insurance, and most of those who do have insurance live in constant jeopardy that the greedy health insurance companies will callously leave them high and dry when they most need care.

Moore's movie brings to public attention the distasteful role of profit motives in shaping the structure and practice of health care, whereas most other civilized societies begin with the premise that access to health care is a basic human right and that the need for care—not family income—should be the deciding factor in health care decisions. Moore compares the United States with France, Canada, Great Britain, and Cuba, and in so doing offers a devastating critique, full of powerful images. For me, one of the most poignant images, one that I will long recall, is of watching the face of a young Canadian whose five fingers were cut off in an accident and who had all five repaired at no out-of-pocket expense because of the universal coverage of the Canadian health care system paid for by income taxes.

The young Canadian listens with a look of bewildered horror as Moore describes the dilemma of an American without insurance who cut off two fingers and was told at the hospital that they could repair his ring finger for $12,000 but that his middle finger would cost $60,000. The American had to choose which finger he could afford to keep and which would become medical garbage. The word my wife Claire used to describe it when we left the theater was "brutal," and I think she is exactly on the mark.

I think back more than a decade to the first Clinton administration, when Hillary Clinton took the lead in trying to reform the American health care system and move it in the direction of universal coverage. I was sitting on an airplane awaiting take off, and a Korean businessman took the seat next to me and started to read the newspaper—the health care debate was front page news. After a few minutes he turned to me and asked politely if I could help him understand something in the newspaper. "Of course," I replied. "My English is good," he said, "but there are two things I don't understand in this article. First, when it says that universal coverage is a 'pie in the sky' idea, what does that mean?" I replied as best I could to explain the meaning of this colloquialism and how in the American political context universal coverage might seem to be so far-fetched as to constitute a "pie in the sky" proposal.

"The second thing," he continued, with a look of concern on this face, "is this. Am I understanding this correctly when it says there are over 30 million people in this country with no health care insurance coverage?" "Yes," I replied. "I think that is the right number." He shook his head sadly and replied, "Don't you care about your people?"

Don't we care about our people? That's exactly the question that Michael Moore's film raises. As I said earlier, there are many strong positive elements in American culture—and Moore mentions some of them in his film (e.g., the volunteer spirit that brought so many selfless helpers to Ground Zero in New York after the 9/11 attacks and helpfulness that so many people show when neighbors are in trouble). These are all true, but there is a powerful socially toxic brew at work in the country that the health care system reveals, a toxic brew that washes over marginalized children at risk.

Fear and brutality are the elements of this socially toxic brew. Over the last four decades Americans have come to be awash in fear, and the events of 9/11 and the subsequent war on terror have only magnified that fearfulness. Politicians have found it expedient to feed this fear—of Communists, socialism, immigrants, nuclear war, terrorism, bird flu. The list of things we are called on to fear is long and ever longer. The mass media conspires with politicians to fuel this fear. One study reports that the more TV people watch the more generally fearful they are.

All this fear mongering allows free rein for greedy and self-interested elites to profit and control. In the health care system it allows self-serving corporations and their political lapdogs to cripple efforts to move toward extracting the profit motive from health care, by spreading the fear that if we make a collective commitment to care for everyone, they will take advantage and bankrupt the system. The result is the brutality documented in Moore's film.

What's this brutality all about? Are we a brutal people? The answer is, as it always is from an ecological perspective, it depends. If you are a Native American standing in the way of America's westward expansion, the answer is a clear yes. If you were an African forced into slavery to maintain the economy of the Old South, the answer is a clear yes. If you are a suspected terrorist undergoing "rigorous" interrogation at Guantanomo Bay, the answer is a clear yes. If you are convicted of murder, the answer is a clear yes. If you are an uninsured individual needing health care, the answer is a clear yes. What do all these situations have in common? Why do they evoke American brutality instead of American caring? They are all about people outside the inner circle; they are all about being part of "them" rather than "us."

The decisive moment in any American public debate is always about casting a group or individual as part of "them." When anyone is part of "them" the dynamics of fear kick in, and the latent brutality in American culture floods the public consciousness. For example, when two boys—11 and 13—opened fire on their school in Jonesboro, Arkansas, in March of 1998, a public opinion poll conducted a few days later found that a majority of Americans favored the death penalty for these two boys. Why? Because the initial reports framed these boys as little monsters, and once they were "them," not "us" the brutal streak took over.

The same thing happened after the Columbine School killings in 1999—when a *Time* magazine cover called them "monsters." It doesn't always happen this way, thank God. When a teenage boy in Kentucky opened fire at his school and killed several people, he was claimed by the community and humane efforts were made to understand and heal him because he was one of "us," not one of "them."

"We" are not monsters—and so long as kids are part of "us" our better angels are likely to prevail. For example, in New York State—among others—the government has voted to provide universal health insurance for kids (figuring the kids are "innocent," even if their parents are not worthy). Americans are generous with their money and time to "good kids" even when they have "bad" parents, but once kids fall from grace they join the ranks of "them," and God help them then. After he had shot and killed his favorite teacher on the last day of school, 14-year-old Nathaniel Brazil faced sentencing. One of the dead teacher's best friends said in public, "I hope he goes to jail and is raped and tortured every day for the rest of his life."

Just how brutal are we to "them?" It was only in 2005 that the U.S. Supreme Court forced us to join the rest of the civilized world in forgoing the barbaric practice of executing minors. Of course, we still execute adults even obviously deranged and/or mentally retarded adults. In a society dedicated to freedom and equality, racism and homophobia still exist in our country and even thrive in the words and deeds of public figures in religion and politics who are allowed to spout their toxic words in many venues without challenge. When we incarcerate kids we still reserve the right to put them in solitary confinement for long periods (e.g., 16 months in the case of one 15-year-old boy I know). The rate of expulsion of children from preschool is three times the rate for high school students according to a Yale University study, because these children evoke fears that they will become so aggressive and antisocial that they will become intolerably dangerous to "us" and our "good" children.

Public opinion surveys reveal that when asked in the 1960s, "Do you agree with the statement that you can trust the government to do the right thing most of the time?" in excess of 80% of Americans answered yes. By the late 1990s, that figure had shrunk to about 20%. Is it any coincidence that during this same period American kids have decreased their general social trust (from 39% of 16 year olds in 1975 agreeing with the statement "Most people can be trusted" to only 16% in 1997). I don't think so. Fear does this.

This declining social trust is toxic because it undermines the sense of "we" rather than "me," which is the other side of excluding "them." We fear that if we care for "them," they will take advantage of us and we believe we must brutally reject that possibility of exploitation. We see this in the current national debate over illegal immigration. The more the immigrants are feared—"They take our jobs." "They bring illness and drugs." "They exploit our public services."—the more they evoke a brutal response.

The Korean visitor who asked me, "don't you care about your people?" hit the nail on the head. There is no doubt that Americans care about their families—and even their neighbors and members of their congregation. Things break down when everyone is included in "we," so there is no "they." So long as everyone is inside the circle of caring our better nature prevails and the American inclination to generosity and helpfulness operate. But once we set someone outside that circle, the dark side emerges, and the rule of brutality prevails. The result is justification for torture (of suspected terrorists, violent young offenders, or for that matter kids who lack health insurance).

Perhaps the other most awful moment for me in Michael Moore's film "Sicko" is when a mother describes in excruciating detail how her 18-month-old daughter died unnecessarily from a high fever for the reason that the hospital to which she was taken would not accept her because her medical insurance would not cover the charges in that hospital. Only the hospital in her policy's network was covered. How brutal is that? American style, that's how. Our fear that mothers (particularly poor, minority, single mothers) like this will "take advantage" of "us" drives the brutality of the way our systems respond. That's what it means to live in a socially toxic environment, and why it can be fatal to kids who have the misfortune to be cast out, to become part of "them."

Chapter 4
The Right to Protection: Child Abuse is the Root of Much Evil

> *Mother: Why didn't you tell the police that I beat you?*
> *Daughter: 'Cause you could kill me.*

One of the fundamental human rights is to be protected from child maltreatment—physical, sexual, and psychological abuse, and neglect. After decades of study it is no longer necessary to spend much time trying to define child maltreatment precisely; I and others have spent enough of our precious time and energy engaged in that task. I will cover this issue briefly.

I have learned that the task of defining child maltreatment is not simply one of listing specific behaviors that fall within or outside the boundaries of the term. No simple list is of much use because there are complex issues of intention (if you hurt a child unintentionally but should have known that what you were doing was dangerous or damaging it is still child maltreatment) and consequence (if you have sex with a child, terrorize a child, or throw a child against a wall and the child is unhurt that does not make it any the less child maltreatment).

More than a decade ago, after having investigated this issue for nearly 20 years, I came to the conclusion that the best definition of child maltreatment is "acts of omission or commission by a parent or guardian that are judged by a mixture of community values and professional expertise to be inappropriate and damaging."

This approach lodges child maltreatment solidly within a human rights framework. It recognizes that protecting children is an ongoing effort to raise the standards for how children are treated as knowledge and awareness increase about what children are entitled to and how that entitlement influences positive and negative development. Thus, at any particular time and place, to label something child maltreatment is to recognize that the institutions of a community have come to understand that the minimal standards of child care are being violated in ways that put the child at risk. Of course, many people find this approach to defining child maltreatment frustrating. They would like a definitive list of what is and isn't child abuse and neglect. But after 35 years in the field I am convinced that there is no such list. There is only a commitment to keep to the task of bringing social and cultural realities in line with our developing understanding of the basic human rights of children: bodily integrity, psychic safety, and nurturance.

J. Garbarino, *Children and the Dark Side of Human Experience.*
© Springer Science + Business Media, LLC 2008

I think of what Michelangelo said when asked how he went about sculpting. Rather than having a precise algorithm, recipe, or set of pre-specified actions, he had a guiding concept and vision. For example, he said, "If asked to sculpt an angel, I take my hammer and chisel, approach the block of stone, and chip away anything that does not look like an angel." Like it or not, that is how we must approach child maltreatment. We must take up our concepts of children's human rights and our understanding of child development and approach the lives of children.

One of the most important consequences of approaching children this way is that we find ourselves drawn to the ways in which the experience of being maltreated can set children off on a negative developmental pathway. It is important to note that the link between child maltreatment is not simple and invariant. Some children exhibit resilience, in the sense that they are not crushed developmentally by the experience of being maltreated in childhood. Of course, even among those who are functionally resilient there may be great sadness and even barriers to a positive inner life and intimate relationships.

Indeed, Michael Rutter's recent review of four studies looking at the consequences of child maltreatment concludes that "a substantial proportion (about half) of all individuals suffering physical or sexual abuse in childhood nevertheless shows unremarkable positive psychosocial functioning afterwards." It doesn't make the violation of the human rights of the maltreated children any less a violation—harm is not the sole criterion for judging maltreatment, after all—but it is good news for victimized children, and indeed for the whole human community.

But what about the children whose development is brought low by the experience of child maltreatment? Although we might consider many deleterious outcomes—depression, sexual dysfunction, economic failure, learning disabilities, physical injury, and death—I am drawn to the role of child maltreatment in setting off a chain of events that leads to problems with antisocial violence and aggression in childhood that become the basis for lifelong problems with antisocial and criminal behavior, what is called conduct disorder in the psychiatric field.

Antisocial aggressive behavior forms the foundation for the diagnosis of conduct disorder—which is just a label recognizing that a child is exhibiting a chronic pattern of aggression, bad behavior, acting out, and *violating the rights of others*. Thus, the violation of human rights that is child maltreatment becomes the basis for perpetuating and extending human rights violation to others. What is it about the way abused kids see the world that leads them to develop conduct disorder? Generally it starts with the fact that they are negative and unrealistic about their social environment.

The social environment is always broadcasting messages, some positive, some negative, and some neutral or ambiguous. Children filter all these "data" through the basic ideas and knowledge they have about attachment and acceptance, and then digest them through their thinking processes (social cognition). Psychologist Kenneth Dodge and his colleagues have found that children differ in how they receive and organize social information, and the results of these differences go a long way toward explaining how conduct disorder arises and flourishes in some children—particularly abused children—and not in others.

Dodge and his colleagues found that the odds that abused children will develop conduct disorder increase dramatically if their thinking about social information is characterized by four distinct patterns in the way they "map" this information: being hypersensitive to negative social cues, being oblivious to positive social cues, having a narrow repertoire of aggressive responses to being aroused, and drawing the conclusion that aggression is successful in social relations.

The first two patterns push a child's social map toward negativity. Under normal circumstances most of us receive both positive and negative social information, and this keeps our social maps balanced, a realistic mix of the positive and negative. This person is smiling, but that one is frowning. This one has a positive tone of voice, but that one has a threatening tone. This one is kind, but that one is mean.

Some kids receive only the positive, and this skews their social map in an unrealistically positive direction—what might be called Pollyanna syndrome—but this is actually more functional and socially desirable than its opposite. The kids Dodge was concerned about suffer from the opposite problem: They receive only the negative and thus see the world in increasingly negative terms. They experience an unrelentingly negative pattern that we might well call a war zone mentality, in which the perception of threat increases and the defensive inclination to hit first and ask questions later arises.

What's more, some of these children are at heightened risk for translating the experience of being victims of child abuse into the experience of being perpetrators of conduct disorder because their understanding of how the world works is also unrealistically skewed. Mark Twain wrote that "if the only tool you have is a hammer, you are likely to define every problem as a nail. "I would say that the reverse is true as well: If you define every problem as a nail, the only tool you need is a hammer."

Kids at risk for problems with aggression suffer from a similar limitation. Their answer to every question is aggression. What to do if afraid? Hit. What to do if confused? Hit. What to do if frustrated? Hit. It is as if they had a road map that had only North on it. All roads lead to aggression; it is the only direction they recognize.

There is more. The problem with these kids is that they have gone beyond simply possessing and demonstrating a narrow range of responses to being angry, afraid, frustrated, and covetous (namely, aggression). They have taken the next step, and actually believe that aggression is successful. It is not surprising that this is a tempting possibility for a child living in an abusive family. Like a little anthropologist, the child observes and records in the notebook of the social map: Mom and Dad are arguing, Dad hits Mom in the face, and she shuts up. Note to self: Hitting works (at least if you can identify with the aggressor). Baby brother is whining for ice cream. Mom slaps him, and he stops asking. Note to self: Slapping is effective (particularly if you are bigger and more powerful than the target of your aggression). I take Billy's toy. He starts to complain to the teacher. I hit him in the stomach, and he shuts up. Note to self: Hitting stops kids from complaining to the teacher if you hit hard enough (and don't get caught).

What is the bottom line in all this? Dodge reports that if, by age six, abused children develop the four risky patterns of thinking (that is, focusing on the negative, ignoring the positive, being limited to aggressive responses, and believing aggression is successful), they are eight times more likely to develop conduct disorder than abused children who don't develop these patterns. Abused children who don't develop these risky patterns of thinking are no more likely than non-abused children to develop conduct disorder; but that raises some very important questions. Why do some abused children develop risky thinking, whereas others don't? Why do non-abused children develop conduct disorder at all? Both invite answers that involve human biology within the child as well as social conditions around the child.

The question of which abused children develop risky thinking and why this happens finds a provocative answer in the work of Avshalom Caspi, Terrie Moffitt, and their colleagues. Their study grew out of research with animals showing that when there was a deficiency of certain chemicals in the brain's (neurotransmitters), the affected animals were more aggressive—particularly when put into stressful situations—because the chemicals involved affected the brain's response to threat and stress. When there is a deficiency of these chemicals, the brain has trouble processing social information effectively in ways that are the animal equivalent of what Dodge and his colleagues demonstrated with children, and these problems lead to more aggressive responses.

Neurotransmitters are under the control of an enzyme linked to a specific gene (monoamine oxidase A, the MAOA gene), and Caspi and Moffitt set out to trace the impact of all this on child development. Through its effect on the enzyme, the gene can turn the important neurotransmitters off—causing the deficiency—or on—leading to normal levels of these chemicals. When the MAOA gene is turned off, the child does not have the same level of activity in the important neurotransmitters of norepinephrine, serotonin, and dopamine than when it is on. The result is that children with the MAOA gene turned off are less able to deal with stressful information and more prone to overreact to potentially dangerous situations.

Does this sound familiar? It should. These are exactly the issues Dodge identified in his study of why some abused children develop conduct disorder, whereas others do not. The results of Caspi and Moffitt's research shed light on the unanswered question in Dodge's research: Why do some abused kids develop risky thinking (and thus become prone to conduct disorder), whereas others don't?

If abused children have the MAOA gene turned off, about 85% develop conduct disorder. If they are abused and have the gene turned on, the figure is about 40%. If the MAOA gene is turned off and the child is not abused, the rate of conduct disorder is about 20%. If the gene is turned on and there is no abuse, the rate is 20%. Although this is only one study, it is consistent with the research on animals. It is also consistent with the body of research demonstrating that the developmental pathways for aggression starts with a nearly universal capacity and inclination to behave aggressively during infancy and early childhood (as demonstrated by the research of Richard Tremblay), but that the processes controlling whether aggression waxes or wanes thereafter are the child's thinking about aggression (cognitive structuring) and his or her experience with aggression (behavioral rehearsal), according to researchers Patrick Tolan and Nancy Guerra.

I think the important conclusion from looking at the intersection of Dodge's research, the findings of Caspi and Moffitt's study, and the perspective brought by Tremblay, Tolan, and Guerra is that the consequences of violating the child's basic human right to live free of abuse are often dreadful, for the child as well as the larger community. The development of conduct disorder in childhood puts children on the fast track for becoming seriously violent delinquents, and eventually adult criminals. About 30% of kids with conduct disorder in childhood end up as seriously violent delinquents in adolescence. Among kids living in violent and antisocial neighborhoods that figure is 60%. Among kids with the MAOA gene turned off that figure is 90%!

This is why the child's right to protection from abuse is one of the most important rights there is: When it is violated the damage can reverberate throughout the lives of individual children to reach the community around them and the next generation of children. We must remember that if we prevent child abuse we can neutralize the relevance of the MAOA gene (that is, non-abused kids with the MAOA gene turned off have no higher rate of conduct disorder than non-abused kids with the gene turned on).

Programs and policies to prevent child abuse do exist. For example, in a program of intervention and research that spans more than three decades, David Olds and his colleagues have demonstrated that home visitors (nurses) who work with high-risk families—pre-natally and then for the first 2 years of life—can reduce the rate of child maltreatment substantially (from 19% to 4% in the original study) and thus prevent subsequent developmental problems, including juvenile delinquency. However, in countries like the United States such programs are not universal.

Assuming that prevention is neither always available nor always effective, there is and always will be a need for treatment services for abused and neglected children. This is the key to effective child protection, because good treatment can break the link between being abused and engaging in a pattern of antisocial violence. Yet, few abused and neglected children receive treatment. (One estimate puts the figure at a pathetic 5%.) I see the bitter fruit of failed child protection every time I enter a prison to serve as a witness in a murder trial, as the following case study makes clear.

Case Study: Untreated Abused Children Inhabiting Adult Bodies on Death Row

Testifying in death penalty cases offers an internship in the destructive consequences of child maltreatment, particularly when coupled with other forms of trauma and deprivation. In case after case I read the records and conduct the interviews, and in so doing come face to face with tales of trauma—physical, psychological, and sexual abuse, street violence witnessed, suffered and perpetrate, gangs, drug dealing, oppression, and racism. It is an awful opportunity to witness what "the accumulation of risk factors" really means to a human life.

Many of my cases are re-trials of cases decided years earlier but sent back to the courts after appeals, so some of the defendants have already been convicted and sentenced to death. As a result, I go to death row for some of the cases, and even visiting is a terrible experience. Some films capture the grim emotional reality of it rather well—two examples being "Dead Man Walking" and the more recent "The Life of David Gayle."

I usually drive out into the countryside to some rural site where the prison is located. I surrender ID, cell phone, and anything that might constitute or hide contraband. Security is usually intense; for example, having a guard watching every moment. Sometimes the condemned prisoner is shackled in front of me in the interview room—hands and feet chained to a post. It's grim.

But what's so hard are not the logistics. What's hard is knowing that I am looking at a dead man (dead man walking) unless I and the others involved in the case succeed in court. What's hard is knowing that I will walk out the door into the fresh air in a short time and the man in front of me will *never* go through that door (since usually the options in the trials in which I am involved are death or life in prison).

What's really hard is hearing the stories of human lives brought so low. The litany of suffering, experienced and inflicted, is emotionally and spiritually grueling. Some of these men have forged a monk-like spirituality out of the crucible of their suffering. Jarvis Master is one, as the tale is told in his book, *Finding Freedom: Writings from Death Row*. But others—most, probably — are demoralized and bitter to the core. When I asked one man on death row what he had learned from 30 years of life, he simply said, "life sucks." I usually swallow and digest this suffering, but not always. One summer several years ago, when three of my cases were coming to fruition at the same time, I traveled to death row three times in less than 5 weeks. After the third visit I spent the time driving back to the airport to return home sobbing. The weight of the suffering was crushing,—and I was just visiting.

Over the years I have heard many stories with the same themes; only the particulars change. What differs is who abused the child, what kind of abuse it was, what the child's injuries were, how soon the child began to come unraveled, what form the breakdown took, and how deeply violence was integrated into the child's strategies for dealing with the world that had dealt him such a raw deal. I always feel like I am sitting with an untreated abused child inhabiting the body of a young man (and in a couple of cases, a young woman).

Let me report on four of these cases: Roger, Charles, Keydrick, and Thomas. Each had committed his capital offense as an adult, but in each case I saw that sitting before me in the interview room was a traumatized child frozen inside the adult man's body. It reminded me of the psychological truth that if untreated, traumatic memories do not decay. They endure for decades, causing havoc to the trapped child.

Although Roger was 42 years old at the time I interviewed him, a full understanding of his actions must take into account his early experiences as a child and adolescent. Roger was born into a dysfunctional family, and this led to him being removed from home and placed in residential facilities until he was 14. Research indicates that early disruption in the mother–child relationship places a child at high risk for later developmental problems, particularly social behavior (including delinquency and criminality). These early experiences were readily classified as child maltreatment, certainly neglect and probably abuse.

In addition, Roger reports experiencing a classic traumatic experience as a young child, witnessing a murder when he was about 6 or 7 years of age. He retains a clear visual memory of this experience but reports no emotional or psychological consequences of it. Given what is known about trauma in young children, this is not indicative of there being no effects, but rather of dissociation and emotional disconnection. What is more, he was placed in residential programs in which numerous forms of abuse were occurring, including sexual, physical, and psychological maltreatment. Additionally, during his youth he had numerous violent and potentially traumatic experiences, such as being shot at. When asked to name the "worst thing that happened to you as a child" he cites, "being sent away from home." When asked about the "worst thing you ever saw as a child," he reports witnessing the shooting.

It is important to note that Roger reports neither the institutional abuses in the settings in which he lived as a young child, nor experiencing psychological consequences of the traumatic experiences he does report (e.g., witnessing the murder). Both the lack of memory and the lack of reported effects are consistent with early trauma. The process of forgetting traumatic experiences and emotionally disconnecting from those for which there is a conscious memory are common adaptations to trauma. His lack of memory does not negate the multiple documentation of institutional abuse, including sexual abuse, in the residential settings in which Roger was placed. They speak to the likelihood that he experienced such maltreatment (minimally that he observed it). He does remember several severe psychological punishments that are reported by others who were residents of the facilities at the same time as Roger.

I believe that these many early traumatic experiences played an important role in shaping Roger's behavior. They were pivotal in his incarceration at age 17 (after just three years out of institutions), his difficulties in prison as a young man, and his involvement in the murder for which he was facing the death penalty. The person before me was a tough 42-year-old man, but inside he carried many untreated traumas, traumas experienced as a young child. In a sense, there is an untreated traumatized child inside the 42-year-old man, and that child's unmet needs have played a powerful role in shaping the experience and behavior of the man. Society was unable or unwilling to protect Roger the young child and the consequences were lethal, as they often are in the case of untreated childhood trauma.

Charles is another example of this. Although Charles is 36 years old, and was 26 at the time of the homicide for which he was convicted, it was his early life that set him on this course. Understanding his life is made particularly difficult because of his difficulty remembering and reporting childhood experiences, which appears to be linked to both the traumatic nature of those experiences and the "family tradition" of secretiveness into which he was socialized. This requires that we lean heavily upon reports made by other family members and by Charles' new emerging ability and willingness to report directly upon his experiences. As Charles says, his mother was like a "CIA director" keeping the family's life as secret as possible; e.g., multiple moves and never leaving a forwarding address, vigorously enforcing her rules that family matters not be discussed or disclosed outside the family, and denying that experiences had ever happened. Charles' loyalty to his mother (which is only now changing as he gains some perspective on her and his early experience) creates another impediment to accessing information about his development as a child and adolescent.

Based upon what is now known, it is clear that Charles was born into a dysfunctional family characterized by highly conflictual and broken relationships as well as high levels of impairment due to substance abuse. He had no relationship with his biological father. He reports that "you never knew who was going to be around" and that "they had no concept of what a family is." As a result of this pattern, care and responsibility for Charles as a child was fragmented and inadequate, including a severely disrupted mother–child relationship. The substance abuse problems of his mother clearly disrupted Charles' relationship with her, as did her extreme treatment of him. These early experiences are readily classified as child maltreatment, certainly neglect and probably abuse.

When asked to describe "the worst thing that happened to you as a child," he reports experiencing a classic traumatic experience, being molested by a drunken adult male "friend of the family." He retains a clear visual memory of this experience, but reports no emotional or psychological consequences of it, which given what is known about trauma in young children is not indicative of there being no effects, but rather of dissociation and emotional disconnection. He was told that the family arranged for this man to be killed in retaliation for this act. Charles reports a vague memory of having been taken to a park to witness this, but is not sure what it is he is remembering.

Charles does say that "every day it was something." He cites incidents such as the ones in which his aunt Gertrude was thrown out of the grandmother's house (for hitting her in the head with a hammer) and was shot at by her lover. He recalls, at age 12, being spanked outside his home by his mother—bare bottom in front of a group of girls. But amidst this sort of traumatic violent experience, Charles cites as particularly painful his Aunts Valerie and Arlene moving away because they were the two people in his family in whom he could confide. This made worse the problems Charles faced in dealing with trauma in a family and neighborhood that generally suppressed disclosure and processing feelings in favor of "being a man."

Charles' family experiences took place in the context of a social environment in which he was exposed to and involved in a high level of violence in the community. He lived in several settings characterized by high levels of gang violence, what are often referred to as war zones. Charles began carrying a gun "for protection" as a result. His maternal grandfather employed a high level of physical and emotional violence as punishment when Charles lived with him.

What's more, it appears that Charles was a temperamentally vulnerable child. He was identified in his family as being "bashful and humble" as a young child. He reports that his mother's homes were always full of unrelated men (usually involved in drugs). He says that "these men with deep voices petrified me." He remembers that as a child liking to listen to classical music and watch ballet. This sensitivity (and presumably his slight stature) led him to being taunted by family and others that "he was going to become a homosexual." It also led to repeated efforts to "make a man out of him" on the part of his mother and others. For example, at approximately age eight, when his mother observed him being bullied (e.g., being hit in the head with a rock) she told him "either you kick that boy's ass or when you come home I am going to kick your ass." Charles says, "I never cried—my mother would not tolerate it." In 1995 when his mother died he reports that he felt "disappointed" but not angry or sad. He says that "I observed and loved my mother." He points to her own difficult childhood and youth (a pattern of abuse and deprivation). He reports his best memory of his mother is "sitting up at night on the sofa sharing a soda and looking out over the city at the stars, just the two of us."

For such a sensitive child, efforts to "toughen him up" are likely to produce a mixture of rage, self-loathing, and compensatory aggressive behavior. Charles says that his mother, grandmother, and uncles were "control freaks." He reports that in reaction, "If I feel that I am being controlled I walk out immediately. I rebelled against being controlled by the gangs or others in prison because I won't accept being put in a feminine role." Charles describes himself as being "like a tea kettle ready to explode." He recalls that smoking marijuana had the effect of "making me more aggressive." The mix of family and neighborhood forces confronting Charles would likely produce just such a contradictory pattern. Charles says, "I have a big grudge against my family." He reports that he was visited by family only once in three years while he was in prison. He only had one birthday celebration during his childhood, and that was a group party with his sisters and wasn't even on or near the date of his birthday.

When he was a child and evidenced interest and talent in drawing, his aunt and uncle offered to send him to art lessons, but his mother vetoed it. Charles says of his family, "Every dream I ever had they stamped out." When asked what he would have become if he had lived in a more supportive family and neighborhood, Charles replied, "an artist." He speaks of how he spent as much time as possible during childhood in his room, "reclusive." This is the focus of his current life in the controlled and isolated environment in which he lives as a prisoner; he is an artist. He says, "If I can't paint they may as well strap me on the gurney."

Keydrick was the victim of severe, pervasive, and prolonged child maltreatment, including physical abuse, sexual abuse, psychological maltreatment, and neglect. In my 30 years as a professional working in the field of child abuse and neglect I have rarely encountered a case equal to this one in its severity and pervasiveness. There is no evidence that Keydrick received any psychotherapeutic intervention to ameliorate his victimization. In addition, at age six, Keydrick witnessed a murder in his home committed by the most significant male adult in his young life. The trauma associated with this experience is itself a significant risk factor, predisposing him to troubled development, socially and psychologically. Once again, there is no evidence that Keydrick received any psychological intervention in response to this horrifying experience. What is more, his mother refused to talk with him about this experience throughout Keydrick's childhood. This denied him perhaps the most important therapeutic resource naturally occurring for children (i.e., emotionally available parents to help children process traumatic experiences).

Keydrick's experiences took place in the context of a neighborhood social environment in which he was exposed to a high level of violence. This high level of violence constitutes what I have identified as an "urban war zone" in my research. For example, a study conducted in Chicago in the early 1990s found that in certain neighborhoods like those in which Keydrick was growing up, 63% of the elementary school children report having witnessed a shooting. This is precisely the percentage found in studies in war-torn Lebanon and among Palestinian children during the peak years of political violence in the West Bank and Gaza strip.

Keydrick's experience of community violence occurred in conjunction with an abusive and neglectful family. These experiences of trauma can affect neurological status and brain development, and thus both emotions and thinking. This combination of biological and psychological trauma creates great risk that a youth (particularly a boy) will develop what I have labeled a war zone mentality. Operating within this framework, the youth views and responds to the world much as a soldier would in a combat zone.

The key elements of this war zone mentality are extreme sensitivity to threat (hypervigilance) and a high probability of responding to perceived threat with aggression. Research on the sequelae of trauma and violent victimization in childhood suggests that the kind of highly impulsive, panicky, and irrational behavior Keydrick exhibited during the two homicides he committed is not surprising, given the severe disruptions of normal emotional and cognitive regulation that can occur to such children, particularly when they do not receive psychotherapy to help them recover.

Although Thomas is 24 years old, a full understanding of his actions must take into account his early experiences as a child and adolescent. Thomas was born into a multi-generational dysfunctional family. He experienced chronic disruptions in caregiving arrangements throughout his childhood, including his mother abandoning him when he was 11 years old. These changes included frequent shifts among relatives due to his parents being physically and psychologically unavailable (for multiple reasons having to do with their substance abuse, mental health, and economic and social problems). These early experiences include a gross lack of care (e.g., being left for 8 hours in a crib during the day and suffering such severe diaper rash as to leave permanent scars and require medical treatment, as well as physical assault with a physical object). He reports that his multiple caregiving experience was so chaotic that sometimes he would not be fed at all as a young child and other times each caregiver would feed him the same meal over and over again. His first memory is of playing with a razor and cutting his lip. It is clear that his experiences would readily be classified as child maltreatment, neglect and abuse, physical and psychological to be sure.

Like many if not most untreated maltreated kids, Thomas has difficulty assessing his family and the deviant way in which he was raised. As he put it, "the way I grew up it's not odd to see family members hauled off to jail by the police." He reports that he often went to the homes of other kids, seeking a more positive environment, and often referred to the adults in these homes as "Mom and Dad."

He suffered numerous early traumatic events in his family. These include witnessing domestic violence, watching family fights, being in a car that was shot at with a shotgun, being hit with a metal pipe by a relative, observing severe substance abuse, and witnessing family members being arrested. He reports chronic dreams with strong traumatic content and themes, such as committing suicide in grotesque fashion.

All this is the bitter fruit of failing to protect children from abuse, failing to protect the most basic human right of all, the right to be safe from physical, sexual, and psychological assault. There literally is hell to pay. For kids who are themselves the product of trauma, to be locked away in adult prisons is a crime in its own right. Does it supercede the crimes committed by these kids? I will leave that to the reader to decide, after weighing the evidence, but I will say that most of the rest of the civilized world considers this barbaric.

And I will say that there is little evidence that trying and sentencing kids as adults does much to make our society safer. And I will say that I find it perplexingly ironic that we give kids adult status as criminals for acting in ways that evidence the immaturity of kids, not the maturity of mind and heart that we normally consider evidence of adulthood. And I will say that we are wasting these kids, some of whom could be significant contributors to their communities if they were healed and reconciled and offered a path of redemption.

Recall the case of Nathaniel Brazil, the boy who shot and killed his teacher in Florida. So what did the judge do in the Nathaniel Brazil case? After I testified about the accumulation of risk factors in the boy's life and offered my assessment of how his life situation affected his state of mind on the day he killed his favorite teacher and after I withstood the prosecutor's onslaught of cross-examination, the judge asked me what I thought should happen to the boy. I told him that first it was appalling and inappropriate that Nathaniel had been tried as an adult rather than the immature child he was. Second, I told him that what he needed was a period of protection and assessment, to find out just how troubled he was and get a better idea of what it would take to rehabilitate him. How long would this take? I supposed that by the time Nathaniel was 18 or 21 the answer might be clear. The judge listened, but replied that the law gave him no sentencing option less than 25 years.

It was a victory of sorts when the judge opted not to impose the maximum sentence of life in prison without possibility of parole, but instead decided upon 27 years followed by 7 years of probation. Nathaniel will go into prison a 13-year-old child, and if he survives, will leave a 40-something-year-old man. This most likely means he will become a savage barbarian, unless through some miracle of circumstances he becomes an imprisoned monk as some others have done.

What have I learned from my visits to the "land of the lost," as one incarcerated youth so eloquently calls it? I have learned to see the child inside the man. I have learned about the durability of untreated trauma. I have learned about how the dark side takes a toll on human development. But I have also learned about the capacity of the human spirit to find a toehold of goodness, even in the bleak world of our prisons. I receive letters from such men from time to time—mostly because they have read my book, *Lost Boys*, and found in it a resonance with the transformation and insight they have experienced.

I have learned that inside most killers is an untreated traumatized child. There are simple monsters on death row—individuals who are so blatantly and thoroughly evil that is it hard to find a shred of the hurt child left (if it ever was there in the first place)—but mostly what is monstrous about the killers I have met is what was done to them and what was not done for them when there was a physical child to go with the psychological child that I see and hear when I interview them. I think it is a measure of our moral and scientific failure that we continue to execute these damaged individuals. As Roger said to me as he sat on death row, "Execution is a shameful way to die."

Chapter 5
The Right to Be Free from Hate: Protecting Voices of Compassion in Times of War and Political Violence

"Mommy, are terrorists people too?"

—Brittany, age 6

One of the most important challenges posed by the "age of terror" and our war against it is the threat that our defensive efforts will erode the best in our culture in favor of the fear-based dark exigencies of "the national security state." For adults there are a series of troubling questions. Will the traditional virtues of American democratic pluralism become subjugated to the imperatives of the war on terrorism, and will this lead to a negative change in American political culture as a whole? Will traditional American liberties be sacrificed to the patriotic imperatives of security, and will dissent become synonymous with disloyalty? These are the aspects of everyday life for adults that are most at risk. But what about children and adolescents? How do the workings of the adult political system translate into the patterns of social life and belief for kids?

Research demonstrates that the political culture of the society they live in can affect the beliefs and attitudes that kids develop. I offer as an example a study conducted 30 years ago by my mentor, developmental psychologist Urie Bronfenbrenner, and me. We set out to study the relationship between the political system in which a child lives and the kind of moral judgments that child makes. From a variety of studies we knew that the moral development of children flourishes in pluralistic social environments. By "pluralistic" we meant a context in which social agents represent somewhat different expectations, sanctions, and rewards for members of that setting. These differences generate conflict that is regulated and moderated by a set of commonly agreed upon ground rules and a common commitment to goals and principles. In contrast, a monolithic (or authoritarian) setting is one in which all social agents are organized around a single set of goals or principles. Conversely, an anomic setting would be one in which there is no integration and common ground, only un-moderated conflict and chaos. Urie and his colleagues had found that families in which both parents have strong and differentiated identities yet share a common commitment to the well-being of their children and to working things out produce the most socially competent and responsible children. Anomic and monolithic families generally produced the opposite result. (This was confirmed by the research of Diana Baumrind on

J. Garbarino, *Children and the Dark Side of Human Experience.*
© Springer Science+Business Media, LLC 2008

"authoritarian" and "permissive" parenting among American families in the 1960s and 1970s.)

In our study, Urie and I were interested in discovering if the results for pluralism in the family would find a parallel in the impact of the political system upon kids' development. We had available at the time data on both the political systems and children's moral judgments from 15 societies. Our focus was on pluralism, defined as the degree to which a society contains and respects diverse social elements in controlled competition for political support, but within a common commitment to democratic values and tolerance.

We used a measure "democracy" developed by a political scientist named Vincent, who studied 91 characteristics of societies and their political systems. The resulting scores ranged from +1.25 to −1.83, with the positive scores indicating pluralism and the negative scores indicating totalitarianism. As it turned out, we did not have any anomic societies to study, so we confined the analysis to a comparison of pluralistic versus monolithic societies. The elements of this scale included items such as "effective constitutional limitations," "freedom of group opposition," "military neutral in political affairs," "free speech," and "current electoral system competitive." We compared the level of "pluralism" in the society to the degree to which the moral judgments of kids in the society reflected a balance of adult versus peer orientation. This was measured through the use of a series of moral dilemmas posed to the children. For example, in one of the dilemmas the child was asked what to do when inadvertently finding the answers to a test in a classroom and being requested by peers to reveal them rather than explaining the situation to the teacher and returning the answers.

In each moral dilemma there was a range of response, from completely adult oriented (e.g., "absolutely certain that I would refuse to go along with my friends") to completely peer oriented (e.g., "absolutely certain I would go along with my friends"). Scores range from −25 to +25, with 0 representing an equal division between behavior urged by peers and adults, and a negative score indicating greater peer orientation and a positive score greater adult orientation. When we compared the scores of kids in relation to the pluralism scores of their country, we found that the more pluralistic a society was the more balanced the moral judgments of its kids (in this case, its 12 year olds).

The bottom line is that the kids' moral dilemma scores in the totalitarian nations averaged 10.26, but for the pluralistic nations it averaged 1.86. Back in 1970, the way 12-year-old kids responded to the dilemma of balancing peer and adult authority mirrored the way the larger society around them handled the challenges of maintaining common goals while allowing conflicting points of view. But note that this study was based upon an historical snapshot.

Back in 1970, some of the countries studied were democratic (for example, the United States, Germany, Switzerland, and the United Kingdom) some were authoritarian, both "right wing" (Brazil and South Korea) and "left wing" (the Soviet Union, Hungary, and Poland). Three decades later, political change has altered the social landscape in many of these countries—most notably in the rise of democracy in Brazil and in some of the former Communist countries, and in South Korea.

Change is possible in the political domain, and we assume, in the world of children's moral development as well. Indeed, other researchers (such as sociologist Glen Elder and his colleagues) have tracked the ways in which the lives of children change in response to political changes such as those that occurred in Eastern Europe after the fall of Soviet Union–style communism and in China after the Cultural Revolution. This research finds that adolescents are most likely to absorb changes in the political culture and incorporate them into their world view in ways that can shape the rest of the adults' lives. When the political system shifts toward democracy and pluralism kids follow suit; but what about when things move in the opposite direction? What about when political threat and violence become the dominant theme? What happens then to the right of children to grow up free of hate?

We face intense challenges to maintain the democratic values of pluralism in the face of threat and fear. Given that the moral development of children reflects these larger political influences we must be vigilant about the education and socialization of children and youth, lest they succumb to the authoritarian threat inherent in the exigencies of the national security state during the age of terror.

In such situations, I believe that the principal threat in the world of children and youth is to the process of moral education, particularly when it comes to the morality of hatred. Research on moral development demonstrates that children and adolescents depend upon adults, and to a lesser degree peers, to stimulate advances in moral reasoning and judgment. This is particularly true in the world of our highest values— justice, tolerance, fairness, and compassion, for example. Children do not develop these values spontaneously. Nor do they apply them in the most sophisticated manner when left to their own devices. No, they need adults who can teach them these higher values and this higher form of moral reasoning through example and discussions that challenge children to move to higher levels of value and reasoning.

The danger I see is that the atmosphere of threat that comes with political violence and the imperatives that come with the national security state will suppress or overwhelm the adult influences necessary for higher moral development. It has happened before. In Northern Ireland, for example, adults in general—and particularly school teachers—were not at liberty to discuss political issues freely, in a way that would stimulate the moral reasoning of their students. Instead, they had to toe the ideological "correct line," or face the prospect of violent reprisal. This is true to a greater or lesser extent in situations of national insecurity around the world. How do we avoid this dark temptation, the temptation to forego compassion in favor of ego, judgment, revenge, dehumanization, and sentimentality?

Christian teaching (among the many spiritual teachings that share its commitment to the higher path—Buddhism, Judaism, Hinduism, and Islam among them) has many texts to guide us in this effort (despite the fact that Christian individuals and societies have often ignored or distorted this guidance). I think some of the best of Christian teaching comes from the Sermon on the Mount. Mathew Chapter 5 records the words of Jesus thus, "Blessed are the meek for they shall inherit the earth."

On the face of it, this may be the most ludicrous truth in the Bible. It is ludicrous because much of the time it seems that the arrogant and power hungry are the ones in charge of the world, not the meek and gentle. This is true, except for the protected spiritual spaces in our lives, such as in church on Sunday mornings, the synagogue on Saturdays, the mosque on Fridays, and the Buddhist meditation room any day of the week, when it seems easy to believe. Ludicrous in the everyday material world, but true nonetheless, because a deeper analysis reveals this to be a profound insight.

A pastor friend much more knowledgeable than I am tells me that "meek" here means "those who have the strength to be gentle." Those who have the strength to be gentle in the face of the material and warring world as it is—often cold, hard, and violent—reach a state of spiritual enlightenment, and nothing is more precious than the bliss and peace this brings.

Enlightenment does not come automatically to children. Children are not always automatically exempt from the temptations of hatred. When I visited Croatia during the tail end of their war with Serbia an 11-year-old boy said of his Serbian enemies, "They are monsters and I hope our army kills them all as they deserve." It doesn't take much imagination to understand how he learned this lesson from the adults in his world—parents, teachers, neighbors, relatives, and politicians—and learn the lesson he did, all too readily.

As I have said earlier, from time to time I testify as an expert witness in murder trials, often involving young men as the perpetrators. I do so usually for the defense at the penalty phase of the trial, where the issue is usually life in prison versus the death penalty, and my job is to explain how the childhood and adolescent experiences of the defendant contributed to his terrible actions. These cases expose me to the darkest sides of human experience, child abuse, rape, addictions, extreme violence, sadness, and despair. But there are lessons to be learned here about how we as adults must become enlightened before we will be able to help children maximize their moral development. As Mahatma Gandhi once said, "You must be the change you wish to see in the world."

I have thought of Gandhi's words often, but never more than in 2001, when I testified in the case of Nathaniel Brazil in Florida (a case to which I referred in Chapter 2). At age 13, Nathaniel committed a terrible murder, shooting his favorite teacher, Barry Grunow, at point blank range on the last day of school in May 2000—a horrible event that was captured on the school's security cameras and broadcast widely on the national news. The murdered teacher was an exemplary human being by every measure, to the extent that in the community of Lake Worth, Florida, where he lived, he was called "the Gandhi of Lake Worth." What finer compliment could a human being receive than to be called the Ghandi of anything.

At the penalty phase of the trial the murdered teacher's friends and relatives were invited to testify as to the effect of the murder on their lives and to speak about what penalty should be imposed. Florida law at the time precluded the death penalty (which at least some of the victim's friends and relatives perceived as a denial of justice). The judge could impose any sentence from 25 years to life. Every friend and relative who testified favored life imprisonment. As I noted in chapter 4, a friend of the murdered teacher was quoted in the press as saying of his support for the boy receiving a life sentence, "I hope he is raped and tortured every day for the rest of his life." The judge sentenced Nathaniel to 27 years.

These were good people. I believe that had they met Nathaniel, heard his sad story before he killed his teacher, their hearts would have gone out to him. Perhaps one of them would have volunteered to be his mentor. But they were unwilling to show compassion to the boy when he committed a terrible act. If you were to look at his life with compassion you would see and hear the story of a troubled boy's life, beset by difficulties. And having heard and seen you would seek to understand and heal him, not condemn to hell on earth. One can easily imagine a similar scenario if Nathaniel had committed a lethal act of terrorism. So what do I think is wrong with all this?

For a start, let's consider the awful irony that Gandhi, to whom the dead teacher was likened, was also murdered (by a Hindu extremist in 1948). We know from all that he wrote and said without a shadow of a doubt what the Gandhi of India would have wanted for the young man who killed him. Yes, he would have wanted him detained to protect the community, but he also would have wanted him understood, healed, and if possible returned to the community in a position to do good deeds as penance for his crime. That the friends and relatives of the Lake Worth Gandhi wanted something different for his killer nearly 60 years later says something important about the social toxicity of American culture and the work we need to do to prepare ourselves as adults to help promote the moral development of children growing up in our care—particularly in times and places of war and political violence.

We need go no further than the acts of terrorism committed by American teenagers and young people to see how our society responds to terrorism. When Dylan Klebold and Eric Harris attacked their high school in Littleton, Colorado, on April 19, 1999, they were engaged in an act of terrorism. They were driven by a twisted world view and motivated by rage. Recall that in the videos they made before the attack they indicated their hope to hijack an airliner and crash it into the World Trade Center. They killed 13 people before killing themselves 2½ years before other terrorists carried out their own plan for an attack on the World Trade Center and killed nearly 3,000 people.

In the aftermath of their attack they were vilified by America. "The Monsters Next Door" read the cover page headline of *Time* magazine on May 3, 1999. Tellingly, when a memorial was created at Columbine High School it contained 13 trees planted in remembrance. A compassionate response would plant 15 trees, recognizing that the two adolescent terrorists died that day as well as their 13 victims, and that the killers were "us" instead of some alien "them." This is the kind of hard work required of compassion, the unwillingness to close out anyone from the circle of caring, no matter what they do in their troubled state of rage and distorted thinking.

I believe that what was being demonstrated in the courtroom in Florida as the court considered the fate of Nathaniel Brazil was the difference between sentimentality and compassion, and it violates the whole spirit of Gandhi's mission on earth. The Dalai Lama teaches that compassion is more than a feeling dependent upon the sympathetic nature of the other. It is the ability to remain fixed on caring for the other person regardless of what that person does, not just out of sympathy for the other person but from the recognition that it is best for ourselves to live in a state of compassion rather than hatred. Jesus certainly recognized this in his life and words.

This does not mean simply ignoring or surrendering to evil, violence, and sin. It means that even in the face of human behavior that is evil, violent, and sinful we still care for the offender, even as we seek to control that person's dangerous behavior and protect ourselves and the community. The understandable sin I witnessed in the courtroom in Florida was the suspension of compassion in the face of rage and hurt, and the substitution of revenge for an ethic of caring. In Christian terms, it is a disavowal of Christ on the Cross calling out to God, "Forgive them for they know not what they do!" And, of course, to simply dismiss the friends and family of the murdered teacher as insensitive seekers of revenge would be to commit the same sin as they did in the courtroom. No, we must love them even as we see the limits of their moral perspective.

Indeed the crucial concept for those who seek to live by compassion, not just sentimentality, is "the circle of caring." The circle of caring describes the area of one's life in which moral values apply; outside that circle the issues are not so much moral as logistical. In the film "Seven Years in Tibet," Heinrich Harrer, an Austrian who comes to befriend the young Dalai Lama, begins work on a building. He arranges for workmen to dig a trench as the start of building a foundation. As they begin work monks approach them and ask them to stop the digging because they are killing the worms. For them, the circle of caring includes even the lowly worm. None of God's creatures is excluded; each creature deserves care and concern.

Every culture struggles with this issue of who is "in" and who is "out" of the circle of caring (and as we saw in Chapter 3, being "out" exposes some of the most toxic elements in American culture). Some of the fiercest warriors in armies throughout history have matched their bloodthirsty ruthlessness on the field of battle with a soft caring for friends and family. Even some of the most monstrous killers may have a small circle of beings for whom they care in a morally elevated fashion. A boy I met in prison had killed several people and would probably kill more if given the chance, but had a special spot in his heart for his pet cat. Hitler had his dog. Even some of the kindest socially constructive citizens have holes in their circle of caring. A loving father and good neighbor attends Ku Klux Klan rallies where he applauds speakers who incite race hatred and bigotry. My best friend in Germany tells me that her loving father who for decades sensitively ministered to the needs of his patients as a pharmacist, to his dying day maintained that if Hitler had succeeded in killing all the Jews the world would be a better place.

The world's great spiritual teachers are at one with Jesus in teaching us to love our neighbors and that everyone is our neighbor, even if the religious institutions stimulated by the lives of these spiritual teachers tell a different story. Historically the Christian church has struggled to expand the circle of caring. In the early years after Christ's death, the issue was, "can the Gentiles be included or is Christ only for the Jews?" During the time of the Crusades "good Christians" went crusading to the Holy Land to slaughter Muslims, and saw no moral problem because these infidels were outside the circle of caring. For many decades in America the issue was race; many White churches insisted that non-Whites were theologically doomed to be "outside" their Christian circle of caring. Today many churches would place gay and lesbian Christians outside the circle—and only "reconciling congregations" seek to include them. Islam has its jihad against "the infidels," including most of the readers of this book, just as some Christians would simply consign Muslim terrorists to hell without a second thought.

The circle of caring must be as big as we can tolerate—and then bigger still. When I testify as an expert witness in murder trials I try to evoke compassion for the murderer by explaining to the court how an innocent child becomes a guilty teenager or adult. Sometimes the opposition seeks to defame and discredit me by claiming, in effect, that I "love" murderers. After the attacks of 9/11, I wrote about the need for compassion as well as action to apprehend those who supported and instigated the perpetrators. The message is that even as we seek to stop terrorism by healing the wounds that spawn it and immobilizing those would commit it, we must not allow ourselves to dehumanize our enemies but rather have compassion for them. Indeed our spiritual teachers would tell us we must love them.

Love the terrorist? I have been accused of that too. Isn't that exactly what Jesus and every other great spiritual teacher calls us to do? Isn't that exactly the message? When the little child asks, "Mommy, are the terrorists people too?" we must be prepared to answer yes. Then we must be prepared to go the next step, "Even though they have done this terrible thing we must try to understand them and help them become better people." No one said being a good Christian, or a good Jew, or a good Buddhist, or a good Muslim, or a good Hindu was going to be easy.

In the wake of the 9/11 attacks many American political and cultural leaders were vigilant in anticipating and attempting to prevent a backlash against Muslims and Arabs in America, and they were largely successful. There was nothing to compare with the racist persecution of Japanese-Americans and Japanese in America in the wake of the Japanese government's attack on U.S. military forces at Pearl Harbor in 1941. But more attacks will make it more difficult to restrain this impulse. After the transit bombings in London in July 2005, police reported that in the 3 weeks following the attacks hate crimes against Muslims increased to more than six times the rate of the same period a year earlier (from 40 to 269). These attacks involved verbal abuse, physical assault, and vandalism aimed at buildings identified with Muslims, including mosques.

Compassion is not just a "value" in the ethical sense. It is a valuable component in the psychological foundations of inner harmony and well-being. There is a parallel here between the way political institutions and individuals respond to the threat of terrorism. On the political level, the "national security state" threatens the values of a democratic society (through intrusions into privacy, torturing terrorist suspects to gain information, and defining dissent as disloyalty). On the personal level, fear and anger can threaten the spiritual well-being of children by virtue of violating the child's right not to hate.

One of the lessons learned from other societies coping with terror and fear origi-nating in political crisis is that efforts to reassure children in the short run can easily poison their souls for the future. For example, in an article published in a social work journal in the 1970s, an Israeli mental health specialist who worked with parents presented a case study of her efforts to help mothers help their young children cope with the deployment of their fathers to the war zone front lines. Here's the essence of her approach: "Remind the child of the time when there was a wasp in the house and his father squashed it with his shoe. Tell the child that there are bad people who want to hurt us and they are like the wasp, and your father has gone out to squash them."

The impulse to demonize and dehumanize the enemy is an understandable response to the challenge of reassuring children in the midst of political conflict and violence. But it does not come without unfortunate side effects in the long run. For example, research from the Israeli–Palestinian conflict reveals that although reassuring in the short run, this approach can impede the process of reconciliation and healing once the political crisis is solved, and it deprives the child of the moral comfort afforded by the world's great spiritual teachings, which universally offer the wisdom of believing in compassion, universal dignity and reconciliation, regardless of whether someone is friend or foe. Compassion is our principal resource in this struggle to maintain our spiritual integrity in the face of worldly temptations to hate and dehumanize our enemies.

Although it is much more difficult to feel true compassion for our enemies, it is essential to achieve a lasting and just peace in the aftermath of military success. It is quite one thing to talk in public about "bringing the perpetrators to justice" and quite another to speak of exacting our revenge. It is one thing to understand the origins of terrorism and anti-American feeling and quite another to portray the struggle as simply one of evil versus good.

Our enemies are typically caught up in their own scenarios of revenge and retaliation. Often they have experienced personal suffering or family loss, or historical victimization, and are seeking a way to give meaning to that suffering through acts of violent revenge. Mostly, they are individuals who are offered a political or ideological interpretation for their situation by their leaders. Sometimes these leaders are pathologically calculating and cold in their exploitation of their followers—as are some of ours. Sometimes these leaders themselves are plotting revenge for what they have experienced as victims of oppression—as are some of ours. For them, the acts they commit are not unprovoked assaults, but rather are their own, sometimes warped version of bringing the perpetrators to justice. We must not fear this understanding. We must not reject those who ask for understanding. We must remember the wisdom that teaches, "if you want peace, work for justice." And remember what Gandhi taught when he said, "You must be the change you wish to see in the world."

The great psychiatrist Harry Stack Sullivan wrote that "people are more simply human than otherwise." What he meant is that we must always seek a *human* explanation for the way people behave, no matter how irrational, demented, or monstrous it seems at first glance. This is an excruciatingly difficult task when the behaviors in question are part of war, political violence, or terrorism aimed at us, our people, but it is essential that we do so for very practical as well as noble reasons.

We may face devastating biological, chemical, and even nuclear attacks in the years to come. How will we make the most we can of these terrible "opportunities" to practice compassion? One place we can look for guidance is the only children on earth who have already experienced nuclear attack, the children of Hiroshima and Nagasaki.

Theirs are the few voices that exist to speak from the ashes of atomic attack. In *Children of the A-Bomb: The Testament of the Boys and Girls of Hiroshima*, Shigeru Tasaka, who was in third grade in 1945 and wrote about his thoughts 6 years later, offered the following proposition:

> For the first time I came to understand what detestable, frightful thing war is…. I think it would have been a good thing if, in the course of this war, atom bombs had fallen on every country…. This is because I believe that by experiencing atom bombs people will understand how barbaric, how tragic, how uncivilized, how hateful a thing war is, and we could have an end of the revolting war we have now." (in Werner, p. 156)

Does the experience of war turn children, youth, and adults against war? As always, the answer is neither yes nor no, but rather, it depends. It depends upon how adults teach children to approach horrible events as opportunities for spiritual insight and the readiness of those children to receive these messages. There are programmatic efforts to teach peace and compassion amidst war and threat. Three American examples are "Project Renewal Post 9/11" in New York City, the Fellowship of Reconciliation, and The Nonviolence Web. Programs exist around the world that share these goals—for example, the M. K. Gandhi Institute for Nonviolence. But are these programs simply imposing a particular set of "values" on the kids who participate in them? How do we decide which values to teach and which to oppose? If we start from an affirmation that *children have a human right not to hate*, answering the question becomes manageable.

One of the challenges faced by everyone in situations of war, political violence, and terrorism is to refuse to be deluded into thinking that we are "pure" and "innocent" victims of whatever the assault may be and that no one has ever faced what we are facing. My experience of the Israeli–Palestinian struggle provides a painful case illustration of this problem, as one of the most contested issues between the two groups is precisely who is entitled to victim status in the conflict. There are lessons here for us.

The first lesson is that the experience of injustice and victimization offers spiritual opportunities just as it offers moral and psychological challenges. What determines whether we seize and grow spiritually from these experiences or allow them to feed the dark side of human selves, our need to be powerful, in control, and angry?

One person who has illuminated the choice we face is psychotherapist and spiritual teacher Dave Richo. Richo has looked closely and with unblinking eyes at how the needs of our egos can push us away from the spiritual opportunities posed by trauma toward the darkness that comes with revenge, anger, and retaliation. He writes:

> Injustice leads to rightful indignation, attempts to repair the abuse, and grief about the loss. Grief is scary mainly because it seems to equal powerlessness. Its alternative, revenge, is resistance to grief, since it substitutes retribution for sadness. It grants a false sense of power because it is power over others, not power for resolving unfairness or transforming human beings." (p. 90)

How does this translate in the world? Richo sees one of its manifestations in the application of the death penalty.

> Capital punishment is an example of a historically legitimized form of revenge. It is rationalized as deterrence. Our wounded ego engages the state to assure we can get even and not have to grieve so ardently or be so much at the mercy of life's conditions. Once we let go of ego, love gains precedence in our hearts and we cannot be satisfied with punishment. We want the transformation of the offender, restitution to us or the community, or the offender's heartfelt restoration to humanity.

He is speaking of "common" criminals, but perhaps the same can be said of terrorists and our reaction to them.

As Americans we are steeped in a culture of sentimentality. We are moved by the plight of victims—whether victims of Hurricane Katrina or the war in Iraq—but only insofar as they remain "easy" victims. But what is our response when victimization leads to a violent response, perhaps a violent response aimed not at the immediate perpetrators of their victimization, but at others in the world who are not at fault, who are "innocent?" Then we are prone to turn our sentimentality into rage and demand revenge, as I explained earlier from the vantage point of my work as an expert witness in murder cases.

What are we called to do in response to those who hurt and despise us? Speaking as both a psychologist and moral philosopher, Dave Richo defines it as "utter reconcilability." By that he means that we must not allow our hurt egos and dark sides to use the opportunity presented by traumatic events to liberate and validate our rage. Rather, we must seek out the greater wisdom of making peace with all and everyone. Every religious tradition and spiritual path offers guidance on this matter. The Christian recipe for divesting ourselves of ego violence and retaliation is in the Sermon on the Mount. There we find the unpalatable recommendations that we turn the other cheek, bless those who hurt us, love those who hate us. In short, reverse every automatic reaction of ego.

Of course religion offers more than just the Sermon on the Mount and the other messages of peace and reconciliation devoid of hungry ego. Most religions also offer a different message as well. For example, fundamentalist Judaism offers the biblical "eye for an eye." Fundamentalist Christianity incorporates this theme and elaborates a retribution model driven by the fires of hell. These are well known to even the casual observer of American life. Judaism and Christianity have a common ancestral link through their relation to Abraham. The third major Abrahamic religion is Islam. Psychologist Scott Gibbs has conducted an in-depth study of Islam from the perspective of humanistic psychology and finds disturbing core support for the kind of judgmental, retributive violence that comes along with Christian and Jewish fundamentalism. The 9/11 conspirators were steeped in this ethos, from a Muslim perspective (which is currently the principal progenitor of suicidal attacks of this sort in the world, but is not the only tradition that can produce such bitter fruit).

The Dalai Lama and Thich Nhat Hanh speak from a Buddhist perspective (one that directly influenced Martin Luther King), and teach that the only way to peace *is* peace, not war or violence. In non-violence the objective is to resolve and reconcile, not gain an advantage. The forces of religious fundamentalism command legions—whether Islamic, Christian, or Jewish (or Hindu, for that matter)—and any effort to seize the spiritual opportunities presented to us by living with political violence, war, and terrorism must come to terms with them, domestically and internationally.

I believe that preparing the next generation of children and youth to do so truly is God's work, the god of love, not the god of war who commands so much of religious history. Remember, religion at its best contains and manifests spirituality, but in some times and places it is subordinated to political power, national interest, and the destructive impulses of egos hungry for revenge against the world.

Pope Benedict XV wrote to the Allied powers at the end of World War I, pleading, unsuccessfully, that they not humiliate the German people. "Remember that nations do not die. They chafe under the yoke imposed upon them, preparing a renewal of the combat, and passing down from generation to generation a mournful heritage of revenge." Judging from the terms of the Treaty of Versailles that ended that war, it seems clear the victorious powers ignored the Pope's wise words.

Two decades later, during World War II, the Soviet dictator Joseph Stalin was asked about how much weight to give Pope Pius XII's opinion. His reply was, "How many (army) divisions does he command?" How many divisions do those with a truly spiritual orientation command in times and places of war, political violence, and terrorism? How can children become members of those spiritual divisions? They can be such only if we protect their human right not to hate. A case study from the Middle East speaks to this.

Case Study: Amidst Hate, a Palestinian Child Speaks of Love

In 1986, I made my first trip into the maelstrom of the Palestinian–Israeli conflict. (I had traveled to Israel once before, but in a way that insulated me from the conflict and absorbed me in a professional experience devoid of much political content.) I traveled throughout Gaza and the West Bank as well as Jerusalem, Haifa, and Tel Aviv as part of a fact-finding mission seeking to understand the issues involved in the Palestinian Intifada, the uprising against Israeli occupation that has continued over the past 20 years, albeit in various mutated forms. The trip took me to the front lines of the Intifada, and was the start of a five-year project to understand the impact of political violence on kids.

In 1986 I visited with kids who were injured in the struggle, injured physically and emotionally, and wrote in my journal:

> How do the kids feel about being wounded? Of course, there is pain and some sadness. But there is also pride in being part of the struggle. They use the word "steadfastness" in the struggle for "the Homeland." There's little expressed rage at the Israelis. There is some use of the term "the invaders." Some of them say, "We want to be free." Their politics bolsters their resolve.

Looking back on it more than 20 years later I'm sure some of this is true. Political meaning does go a long way to make psychological sense of physical injury. I hear that about every conflict, every war. I have said it myself in comparing the impact of trauma in the "senseless" violence of the inner city gang wars to the "meaningful" wars of liberation around the world and between countries. Twenty years later

I would hear it about suicide bombers, and some of the kids I met in the hospital in Gaza may well have become the suicide bombers of 2002. They represent heroism and martyrdom, the ultimate sacrifice in the name of "the cause," certainly for those left behind. But I wonder now about whether this political meaning is really enough for the injured kids.

I particularly return to a 10 year old who was shot in the stomach, the one whose picture sits on the wall of my office to this day. There is so much rhetoric, so many euphemisms, too much rationalization. I don't know this boy, but over the years that followed my fist visit to Palestine I listened to others, younger and older, mouth the language of political struggle. Mostly they are neither better nor worse than the adults around them, on every side around the world. But when it comes right down to it, the physical realities of violence are here in this boy's face.

I was deeply moved years ago by what one soldier said after he had been in battle. When asked, "What's it like?" he replied, "It's not like anything, it just is." An Israeli friend of mine who has lived through three wars and has been decorated twice for his heroism says that he only began to understand this during the 1973 war when he said goodbye to a friend as his boat left shore to cross the Suez Canal, and then 2 hours later recognized his friend's boots coming ashore, sticking out from the shroud that covered the rest of the body. It was then, my friend says, that he understood completely that no sane person who knows war could want to go to war. This is what I saw in the eyes of the 10-year-old boy lying wounded in the Gaza Hospital.

In Chapter 2 I wrote about "Snowden's Secret," as one of the dark secrets kids—and adults—learn from encountering violence first hand, learning that the human body is so fragile that even belief in "the cause" does not dispel the pain and the horror of what bullets can do to a human body. It was there in that hospital in Gaza that I first embraced this concept, an understanding that has sustained me in the years that have followed. It is a dark lesson learned over and over again in all the political violence of the world before and the world to come.

Every war zone demands that we make choices, one of them being whether or not to give in to the temptation to hate. I hold on to one saintly little girl I met first in 1989 in the Jalazon Refugee Camp outside of Bethlehem. Fedwah was then 10 years old. I met her and her family on a tour of the camp in which I had a chance to interview children, often asking them to draw pictures and then comment upon them. There were many fascinating and disturbing stories told, but no child captured my heart as did Fedwa. The oldest of four children, she told me she wanted to help her people when she grew up. Her mother told me that the little girl had set up her own school to teach the younger children because the regular schools were closed due to the conflict. The translator asked if she wanted to be a teacher. "No," she said. "I want to be a doctor."

Fewa's drawing was a scene I had come to recognize readily: Israeli soldiers, checkpoints, children sent home from school because it was closed, a rock-throwing demonstration, children waving the banned Palestinian flag, burning tires. "How are the children feeling?" I asked her. "Enthusiastic," she replied. "How do the soldiers feel?" I asked. "They want revenge against the children because of the disturbances and they feel frightened because they might be hurt," she answered. She told me that the soldiers come into the camp at night, sometimes coming into her house.

"Are you afraid when the soldiers come?" I asked. "No," she said proudly—after all, she is a grown-up 10 year old. "But the little children are afraid," she volunteered. "What do you do then?" I asked. "I try to comfort them," she said. "How?" I asked. "I explain to them that the soldiers are human beings like us. They do this because they have orders, but when they go home they are good fathers to their own children, gentle and kind." Amidst the terror and anger and conflict and hostility here was a little saint, a girl who embodied everything I myself aspired to be as a spiritual person. She refused to accept the easy path of dehumanization of her enemies. Her "revenge" would be to become the best possible person she could be to contribute to the cause of her people. It was humbling, then, and in the remembering still is.

It provided a vivid personal illustration of something my colleagues and I found in our research on how Palestinian kids made sense of the political violence around them. In our study we found that kids fell into three groups: one that expressed passive victimization and defeat (whose images were of hopelessness and despair), one that expressed the desire for violent revenge (whose images emphasized taking up arms for violent struggle), and one that expressed a commitment for positive struggle (whose images put at the center the desire to develop skills and resources that could be used to advance the development of their people). When we looked at the mental health scores of the three groups, the passive victimization group was least healthy, followed by the armed revenge group. The healthiest group was the one that espoused positive struggle. My friend and colleague Jim Gilligan always says that violence is "demented." I agree, and the evidence from these Palestinian kids validates that view.

I visited Fedwah several times in the years that followed that first visit in 1989. I saw in her the promise and despair of the conflict between the Palestinians and Israelis. Year by year I saw her profound decency and humanism challenged and eroded by the waves of oppression, violence, duplicity, and escalating extremism that washed over her community in its struggle to realize the Homeland.

I lost touch with Fedwa in the mid 1990s, but think of her often. In my best dreams she continues her saintly pursuit of a truly humanized response to the conflict. Perhaps she did become the doctor she aspired to be in 1989 and is healing her people. In my heart, however, she is still the little girl in the picture on my office wall, the little girl with my arm around her shoulders. In my worst nightmares her altruism has been captured by the dark side of the Palestinian martyrdom and escalating fanaticism in the face of Israeli oppression and intransigence. I trembled when I read of the first female suicide bomber in 2002, a gentle young idealistic woman who was so committed to the struggle that in her frustration and pain from the losses suffered in her community gave her life and took others in one final effort to teach something profound.

I know it wasn't Fedwa, but I fear it could have been. She was pure and deep enough, and the history surrounding her life hateful enough to drive any sensitive person crazy enough to do such a thing, not out of rage, but out of sadness and commitment to the higher purpose of her people and their homeland. If her human right not to hate was violated again and again in the dehumanizing rhetoric of hate that has escalated in the years since I met her in the Jalazon Refugee camp perhaps she succumbed. After all, she was "only" human.

Chapter 6
The Right to Be Economically "Regular": What It Means to Be Desperately Poor

Poverty is the worst form of violence.

—Mahatma Gandhi

What are the human rights of children with respect to the economy? While we might concern ourselves with a range of issues, from being protected from exploitative advertising to being protected from abusive child labor, this chapter focuses on "What rights do children have when it comes to poverty?" Without diminishing or trivializing any of these other issues, I focus on poverty because it an issue of global importance and one that is of preeminent importance in the lives of children around the world.

When I think about poverty, many images flood into my consciousness. I think of all the poverty-stricken children I have met in the United States and around the world. Their faces fill the pictures that line my office walls, just as their stories haunt my memory. Children living in squalor in Brazilian slums. Children playing in open sewers in Guatemala. Children starving in Sudan. Children living in dilapidated public housing projects in Chicago. But I always come back to my mother's life as a poor child in England in the 1920s and 1930s as an anchoring point.

My mother's family did not starve and they had clothes on their backs, but they had few material possessions, and more importantly, they lived on the edge of economic disaster. And it took its toll: One of her siblings and both her parents literally died from the accumulated stress of living in poverty. She tells many stories of what it meant to be poor in England in the 1930s, but one of her memories of growing up poor touches me particularly.

She recalls being sent by her mother to the local money lender to borrow enough money to feed the family's children until Friday when her father got paid. More than 70 years later she still feels the shame of it. It was not the simplicity of the material conditions of her childhood that was the problem. It was the social threat, the psychological vulnerability and shame she felt. I don't think children have a right to be rich, but I do think they have a right to be free from economic shame, to know that they have the basics for a decent life in their society, to feel they are *regular*.

In North America, as in the rest of the world, families with young children are more likely to be poor that other segments of the population. This was not always

J. Garbarino, *Children and the Dark Side of Human Experience.*
© Springer Science+Business Media, LLC 2008

true in our country. Prior to the 1960s, the poverty rate for the elderly exceeded that for young children, but a massive social intervention changed this—effectively weakening the link between being old and being poor. This is an important model for us. It is a fundamental matter of public policy—and thus implicitly if not explicitly a matter of human rights—that vulnerable categories of the population be protected from the "natural" workings of the economic system.

What does it mean to be poor? In one sense, this question is easy to answer: Government agencies and non-governmental organizations around the world compute numerical definitions that set cut-off points going up and down the economic ladder. In the United States the most common numerical definition is about $19,000 per year—$52 a day—for a family of four. Globally, the focus is on the extreme poverty represented by families existing on $1 or $2 per day—$365 or $730 dollars a year. There are a bit more than two billion children in the world. Half live in poverty of this sort. Organizations like GlobalIssues.org collect and report these data.

Being poor means being at statistical risk. Poverty early in life is a special threat to development, at the most basic level because it can compromise a child's biological and psychological systems. Research tells us that poor children live in the kind of environments that generate multiple threats to development, threats that lead to high rates of academic failure, maltreatment, and learning disabilities. Around the world (according to UNICEF), some 30,000 children die each day due to poverty— like my mother's sibling. That's 210,000 per week and 11 million per year. They die because they lack access to basic sanitation, health care, and adequate food, and experience other toxic factors that can be linked to poverty.

That is one clear meaning of being poor in any society that allows the state of children to be highly correlated with the economic status of that child's family. If society allows it, being poor exposes children to more physical toxicity as well. Around the world, low income populations are more likely to be exposed to chemical and radioactive waste and polluted air and water. But these toxic factors can be un-linked through social policies and programs that assert and support the human rights of children.

How does that "un-linking" happen? In Canada it has meant providing a real safety net of social and health services for poor children (policies and programs often presented as human rights issues). As a result, for example, when we compare the results of research in Canada assessing the strength of the link between poverty and child abuse with similar research from the United States (where the safety net is not viewed as a human right, and thus access to basic care is always conditional) we find the link is stronger in the United States than in Canada. In statistical terms, this means the correlation between the demographic and economic indicators of poverty and rates of child maltreatment is higher in the United States than it is in Canada (or at least it was when the research was done in the 1980s and 1990s).

In Brazil, under the leadership of President Luiz Inacio Lula da Silva, one form of the effort to un-link poverty from toxic conditions for children started in 2003, as a government campaign called "Zero Hunger." The idea was simple. As President da Silva put it, "We are going to create the conditions so that everyone in our country can eat a decent meal three times a day, every day, without needing donations from anyone."

Of course, from the perspective of the basic human rights of children this access to three meals a day should be part of a larger commitment to the proposition that basic education and essential health care should not be dictated by a child's parents' income. Four years later, Brazil's campaign has not achieved its goals fully, but the commitment to address the human needs and thus the human rights of the poor is clear: In 2006 the national spending on social assistance, food security, and income transfer were US$11.3 billion, with the Ministry of Social Development and Fight Against Hunger serving over 60 million people according to federal government reports.

The starting point for any discussion of the economic rights of children is always this same issue, i.e., whether a society will mobilize its resources to shield children from the economic consequences of their parent's economic success or failure. The next step is to see how extreme poverty is fundamentally a human rights issue and how approaching it from that perspective is the key to eradicating poverty and thus nurturing children.

Two world-renowned economists (Jeffrey Sachs of the Earth Institute's Millennium Villages Project and Grameen Bank's Muhammad Yunus) seek to eradicate poverty through a massive global intervention that goes beyond the traditional mix of the infrastructure to support economic activity and job creation and capital accumulation. What is the essence of this intervention? It is to implement a basic human rights campaign as a means for stimulating economic growth among those in extreme poverty—the one billion people worldwide who live on $1 per day.

Although not explicitly conceived and promoted as a human rights campaign I believe these efforts are best thought of in these terms. The key is that Sachs and Yunus do not focus on "abstract" human rights—the rights to free expression, political independence, legal due process, and so on. Rather, they focus on the human rights issues that are paramount in the context of extreme poverty—the concrete basic human rights to be free from hunger, have drinkable water, be free from debilitating disease—and while they're at it, to help them have sufficient credit resources to have access to some small means of production (like more productive seeds and fertilizer for impoverished farmers and tools for village women workers). Sachs and Yunus advocate for meeting these human rights challenges not as an end unto itself, but as a means to promote economic development that will eradicate poverty.

In his book, *The End of Poverty*, Jeffery Sachs shows how this approach flows from an analysis of why people are extremely poor, namely, that they are too sick, weak, and hungry to be very productive. It makes sense. And it makes particular sense that in this state parental ability to meet the developmental needs of children tends to be quite limited. Basic economic development of the sort envisioned by Sachs and Yunus can thus benefit infants and young children both directly (by increasing their nutritional intake and access to basic care) and indirectly (by improving the role models presented to children by their parents).

But will these efforts succeed in eradicating poverty and thus improving the development of infants and young children? I doubt it, because there are so many political leaders who have self-interested agendas, because there are so many sources of violent conflict that can and will disrupt efforts to promote the basic human rights to which the program is directed, because the developmentally hobbling traditions of many local cultures in many areas of extreme poverty (like patriarchal-based oppression of girls and women) will get in the way, because issues of global warming and climate change will undermine the effectiveness of many local community interventions, and finally, because too many people are too self-involved and preoccupied to support the effort in the long run.

What conclusions do I draw from this? The most important one is that despite the built-in impediments to Grameen Bank, the Millennium Villages Project, and other efforts that adopt the same model, I believe that Yunus and Sachs are correct in their analysis and their strategy, and they will help protect many children from poverty. What is more, these interventions and any others that parallel them are the *only* efforts that will do anything substantial to reduce the fundamental violence of human rights that is extreme poverty. Traditional capital-intensive infrastructure projects are of only limited value when they do not accompany the micro-enterprise and health programs envision by Yunus and Sachs. But there is more to this than simply increasing economic assets for the very poor, particularly if our concern is the welfare and development of infants and young children.

When Gandhi said that poverty is the worst form of violence, he was on the mark. When Thich Nhat Hanh said that there is no way *to* peace, because peace *is* the way, he was absolutely correct. And when Sachs and Yunus say that only by mobilizing an intervention to guarantee the basic human rights that extreme poverty violates can there be economic peace they are also exactly correct.

We will return to this at a later point, but first we must take a closer look at how poverty manifests in the social and psychological lives of children, what it means to their minds and hearts. Being poor is about being left out of what your society tells people they could expect if there were included. This is relative poverty. At root, it's a social issue, an issue captured for me in a question a kid asked me at the conclusion of the interview I was conducting with him as part of a psychological assessment. He asked, "When you were growing up were you poor or regular?"

That's it precisely, Are you poor or regular? Being poor means being negatively different; it means not meeting the basic standards set by your society. It is not so much a matter of what you have as what you don't have. It means being ashamed of who you are—and that in and of itself can be an instigator of violence toward self and others as well as a host of other negative developmental trajectories.

There are limits to the social-psychological definition of poverty as an experience of "relative deprivation," however. The young daughter of a colleague of mine once wrote in a composition for school that she was poor—in fact "the poorest kid on the block"—because she lived in the smallest house on the block. She did indeed live in the smallest house on the block. However, it was a seven-bedroom house on a block of even larger mansions. What does it mean to children to be poor if their standard is that being poor is simply having less than others, without any anchoring of the adequacy of what those others have?

If poor children around the world are shoeless, how do we make sense of U.S. poor kids wearing $150 running shoes? In China, an old man once reported to me that before the 1948 revolution very few people were rich, but now (this being 1982) many people were rich. As evidence, he pointed to the fact that he himself owned a wristwatch, a radio, and a bicycle. By that standard poverty is virtually absent in the United States, and we Americans are nearly all rich. Of course, 25 years later, I doubt the man I met in China in 1982 would consider himself rich with only those three possessions. In the new affluent China, a car, a television, a computer, and a cell phone would probably be a more psychologically realistic measure of being "rich."

When most people around the world live on incomes of a few hundred dollars a year, what does it mean to define the U.S. poverty rate at $19,000 a year for a family of four? In some analyses, India has defined poverty as having access to less than 2,100 calories per day and, using that yardstick, estimated that 20% of the population are poor (a figure roughly the same as ours in the United States). Certainly our concern with the human rights of children cannot mean simply endorsing the unending upward spiral of materialism, the arms race of getting more and more things.

There is no human right to be rich! There must be more to it! The human right at stake is to be regular *and* we must wage an unending struggle to anchor children (and parents) in a concept of basic needs that goes beyond simple insatiable materialism to rest upon a sound foundation of spirituality, community, and meaningfulness. But we cannot forget that for a billion children the issues really are those of the most basic right to be "regular," namely, to have water to drink that will not make you sick, to have enough food to eat so you don't go hungry, to have shelter enough to stay warm and dry, to go to school and receive basic health care, and most important of all, to feel economically secure. These are the basic criteria for being "regular."

However, in the modern world, the irregularity of the poor is ever more blatant. Many first-person accounts of life in an earlier era seem to say, "I didn't know I was poor until...." For example, a priest of my acquaintance tells the story of spending a day at school putting together "poor baskets" for Christmas, only to be shocked the next day when one was delivered to his house. "I never knew we were poor until that day," he recalls. I suspect the odds that a child today would be oblivious to his family's poverty are much reduced because images of affluence abound through the mass media and its advertising messages.

Poverty sends messages of shame, perhaps more now than ever before. Why? Because more and more of daily life is under the control of dollar transactions ("monetarized" to use a technical term), and as a result the poor are ever more marginalized—and thus shamed for their irregularity. There are two economies at work in our society—and increasingly in every society in the world.

Mom feels your head and says you feel hot, so she takes your temperature and sends you to bed early because you are coming down with a cold. Dad tells you to wash your hands before you come to the dinner table. Grandma takes care of you while mom's at work. Dad sits with you in the morning until the school bus comes.

Your older brother fixes your bicycle and repaints it. Your sister's backyard vegetable garden yields tomatoes for dinner and flowers to bring to your teacher. The man next door shows your dad how to fix the leaky gutter on your house. Your mom shows his wife how to repair a hole in her sweater. The kids down the block put on a puppet show in their back yard. You organize a ball game in the street in front of your house. All this presents a great deal of economic activity—"transactions of goods and services"—yet all of it is invisible to conventional economic accounting systems. None of it appears in the Gross National Product (GNP); as far as traditional economics are concerned its value is $0.

What will it take for these goods and services to appear in the GNP? Consider an alternative scenario. Mom drives you to the HMO office where the nurse uses a disposable plastic thermometer cover ($2) over the electronic thermometer ($75). The home health video sent home from school ($19.95) admonishes you to use disposable antiseptic moist towels ($.75 each) to clean your hands before each meal. Dad drops you off at the child care center ($10) on his way to work, from which you are bused to school later and then are returned after school for a couple more hours ($20) until Mom can pick you up. Your older brother helps you bring your bike to the repair shop to be fixed and repainted ($56). Your sister picks up some tomatoes ($2.75) and flowers ($5.95) at the store on her way home from school. The neighbor refers you to a good roof repair service to fix your leaky gutters ($375), and your mom tells his wife about the clothing repair service at the local cleaners who can fix her sweater ($10). The kids down the street invite you over to watch the Disney Channel on cable TV ($45 per month) and in return, you let them play your new video game ($32.95). Total contribution to GNP: $655.35.

What all this comes down to is that the GNP measures the cash transactions involved in goods and services that take place in a society; it measures the monetarized economy. The GNP does not measure the non-monetarized economy, because activities don't count if no money changes hands. The economic story of the past 50 years—globally as well as in the United States—has been in part the shifting of goods and services from non-monetarized to monetarized economies. For example, according to some estimates, until recently more than 90% of basic health and child care activities were conducted in the non-monetarized economy. But now monetarized health and childcare are multi-billion dollar enterprises in most "modern" societies. What is more, much of what was once "free" or "for the common good" has become privatized, which means that only those who have cash have access and can participate. The irregularity and marginality of the poor increases as monetarization proceeds.

All of this conspires to make poverty more evident and more shameful. It puts more pressure on parents to generate income and in so doing accentuates the human costs of being poor. If you lack cash in a monetarized society you will feel poor, because you will not be able to have many of the pleasures and necessities of life. And in so doing, monetarization promotes a social climate that violates the human right of children to feel "regular."

In a non-monetarized economy, transactions involve mutual and reciprocal services—and time, of which everyone starts out with an equal supply. If you have access to a strong non-monetarized economy you may not feel poor even though you lack cash—at least if no one rubs your face in the fact that you are not a player in the monetarized economy and then judges you negatively for that.

This analysis of the dynamics of the monetarized versus non-monetarized economies sheds important light on the issue of poverty, in part because as monetarization proceeds it tends to exacerbate economic inequalities. The non-monetarized economy tends to be fundamentally egalitarian because everyone has equal time and everyone has some talents to share (even if it is just your presence). But in the monetarized economy the value of people's time tends to diverge, and that variance has accelerated in the modern era. Those at the top *are* more valuable than those at the bottom precisely because they can generate so much more money.

Concepts like "opportunity cost" attest to this. Opportunity cost refers to the difference in dollars earned from choosing to invest one's time in "productive" activity (e.g., putting in an hour working) versus "non-productive" activity (e.g., attending your child's school play). All of this compounds the issues of economic inequality, with their attendant social implications, both within and across societies. Globally, the data indicate growing economic (i.e., monetarized) inequality among societies as modernization has moved forward. Wealth is possible in dramatically different ways since the advent of technologically driven monitarization, and an analysis of long-term trends presented in the 1999 Human Development Report from the United Nations Development Program reveals that the gap between rich and poor countries (expressed as the ratio of wealth in the richest to wealth in the poorest) has grown since the early 1800s:

- 3 to 1 in 1820
- 11 to 1 in 1913
- 35 to 1 in 1950
- 44 to 1 in 1973
- 72 to 1 in 1992

Analyzing the meaning of poverty for children is not simple. It is not a matter of simple accounting. Rather, it calls for thinking about the relationship between the meaning and meeting of basic human needs and the social conditions that shape those meanings. In one sense, we could solve the poverty problem in the United States by simply adopting the Indian standard (almost every American has access to 2,100 calories per day)—or indeed any of the many measures of poverty used globally (almost everyone in the United States has at least a dollar or two per day)—except one, perhaps, the measure of income inequality.

There are several approaches to measuring economic inequality. The Luxembourg Income Study compared the ratio of incomes for the top 10% of the population with that of the bottom 10%. These comparisons were made after taxes and income transfers are taken into account (because a society's economy may generate inequality but its political system can seek to reduce that inequality by income redistribution programs that supplement the incomes of the poor directly and/or fund public services such as education, health care, and recreation so that family income becomes less of a factor in children's quality of life). Using this approach, the study revealed that among industrialized "rich" countries, the United States had the worst ratio—about six to one—whereas Sweden had the best—about two to one (with Canada at four to one and no country other than the United States above four to one).

Other research (such as that published by Corporate Watch's 1997 report, *The Corporate Planet*) has validated this result: Among modernized industrialized rich countries, the United States has a high degree of income inequality. One of the important statistical measures of this inequality is the Gini Index. It compares a country's divergence from complete income inequality (i.e., if each 10% of the population receives 10% of the income the Gini score would be zero and if the top 10% controlled all the income it would be 100). Scandinavian countries usually report the lowest Gini indices (e.g., Denmark's score is 24), and most industrialized nations have scores of about 30. The worst countries (i.e., the countries with the most inequality) have scores of about 70 (e.g., Namibia's score is 71). The United States has a score of about 41.

Getting directly to the matter of the lives of children, we can turn to infant mortality as one of the best simple indicators of the material quality of life in any society. Usually expressed as the number of infants per 1,000 live births who die before their first birthday, the infant mortality rate says a great deal about how well communities are doing in meeting basic human needs, particularly health and nutritional needs. Why? Because without un-linking interventions it is correlated with poverty and the unavailability of medical technology that comes with being poor unless a human rights–based social policy intervenes.

Infant mortality directly reflects the political priorities of a society. Societies with equal resources sometimes have very different rates of infant mortality (despite the fact that in general, wealthy countries have lower rates than poor countries). On the whole, the number of babies who die reflects a society's willingness and ability to marshal its resources on behalf of its next generation. A highly motivated community can lower infant mortality significantly without fundamentally altering the socioeconomic order by providing good maternal/infant care, prenatally and postnatally. Being born to a poor family need not be a death sentence for a baby.

In the United States, for example, between 1920 and 1980, infant mortality decreased from about 80 per 1,000 to about 12 per 1,000 (the figure was double that for non-Whites) due mainly to improved public health measures and provision of maternal-infant care. By 2003, it was under 10 per 1,000. The world leaders on this score post figures of about 4 per 1,000, but anything 10 and under is good by international standards.

But infant mortality goes up in times of deteriorating social and economic conditions for families, particularly for families otherwise at risk, such as unmarried teenagers and large, low-income households. In the United States, as the recession of the early 1980s deepened, infant mortality rates began to creep up in the areas hardest hit by economic disintegration. This did not occur from society's lack of wealth during this period, but rather from the way wealth was accumulated and distributed.

This paralleled a global pattern. During the period 1980–1998 as the global economy flourished, progress in reducing infant mortality around the world slowed considerably when compared with the previous two decades, when more societies were committed to social progress rather than simply fitting into the emerging global economic machine—often as dictated to them by institutions such as the World Bank.

In Brazil, for example, the boom years did not produce dramatic improvements in the infant mortality rate commensurate with the growing total wealth of the society. The officially reported rate was about 80 per 1,000 for the richest, most developed of Brazil's states such as Rio de Janeiro, and reached 130 per 1,000 in the poorer states such as Bahia. It appears that overall, the Economic Miracle may even have led to increased infant mortality in Brazil because it disrupted the economic and social foundations of the large rural population while creating massive and unhealthy urban slums where services were mostly non-existent and health and social conditions were extremely harsh.

Among the tens of millions of poor families, hundreds of thousands of children were dying in their first year of life in Brazil. The rest were living to face an uncertain future as refugees in the economic war. Brazil presents an important case study of how the human rights of children may suffer because of poverty.

In the 1960s, American comedian Jackie Vernon joked that when President Johnson declared his "War on Poverty," he (Vernon) "went out and threw a hand grenade at a beggar." One of the distressing things about life in the twentieth century was that it seemed all the macabre jokes eventually came back at us as news stories. The surreal character of so much of what passes for public policy becomes the grist for the comedic mill.

"Throwing a hand grenade at a beggar" as part of the war on poverty hardly seemed out of the question in the global economic war that raged in the latter part of the twentieth century (and continued into the twenty-first century). With police and soldiers in Latin America and elsewhere opening fire on protestors in food riots, executing street children, and assassinating dissidents who gave voice to the poor, Vernon's macabre joke became a news item.

Writing from Santiago, Chile, for *The Nation* magazine, Marc Cooper quoted a priest working in the slums as remarking, "The only economic miracle here is the fact that so many people still find one way or another to feed themselves." But at what cost? And at what cost do the rich sleep at night with full stomachs? Poverty is hardly ennobling, particularly in a society in which the contrasts between rich and poor are reinforced daily in the mass media. Brazil provides a compelling illustration.

Case Study: The Morally Destabilizing Effects of Poverty in Brazil

Brazil was the largest and most populous country in South America when I first visited in 1983. It still is. If it is known at all to geographically challenged Americans, it has been known as the site for the sexy Carnival in Rio de Janeiro. More recently, Brazil is known for being a country that weaned itself of foreign oil dependence through a massive bio-fuels program. With more than 180 million people, it is the sixth largest country in the world. But many people who know it well say that because of the enormous income inequalities in Brazil (its Gini Index was about 58 when I landed there for the first time in 1983), it is more realistic to think of Brazil as two very different nations within one country.

One is affluent and totally modern; the other desperately poor and backward. Some commentators have suggested that the best way to think of Brazil is as the countries of Belgium and India existing within the same official political boundaries. To get the numbers right, we might do better to have spoken of "Bangladesh inside Canada," the modern affluent society of some 25 million controlling a vast rich land in which some 105 million desperately poor people live with little hope of gaining access to that wealth.

In 1983, the population of Brazil was 130 million, with more than 65 million 15 years of age or under. Of these kids, some 20 million were considered "abandoned" by UNICEF. Twenty million! A whole country's worth of kids on their own—on the streets with little or no ongoing supervision by adults in families. It was a staggering number to contend with, emotionally, intellectually, and morally. I had my first encounter with some of these abandoned kids within hours of landing in Rio. After settling in at the hotel my companions and I set out to test the surf at Ipanema Beach.

While we were on the beach at Ipanema, a group of young thieves who appeared to range in age from 11 to 15 swooped down on our towels and clothes, taking our two volunteer guards by surprise and running off with whatever money and valuables were to be found. We were lucky visitors: The lesson was learned cheaply because there was little there to be taken. We doubled our guard and successfully defended our property for our remaining time on the beach.

As we were leaving the beach at Ipanema, however, we witnessed again what many Brazilians were calling the "informal income redistribution" system. A youth ran by us before we could register that he was fleeing from a man who shouted, "Ladrao!" (thief!) as he pursued. In what seemed almost a ritual of negotiation, the young thief first dropped the man's ID, then his credit cards. The pursuing victim first slowed, then stopped as he retrieved this critical part of his stolen property. The bargaining completed, the thief ran off unmolested, as much as to say, "I have the money and the wallet; you have the rest, fair enough?" It almost seemed so, this informally negotiated income transfer between one of Brazil's "haves" and one of its "have nots" accepted, if not embraced enthusiastically by the "donor." Most likely, the youthful thief had been one of the abandoned children, and now had graduated to adolescence. We must always remember when looking at teenagers like him that for the most part, adolescence represents more an intensification of childhood issues than it does a change of developmental direction, more of the same rather than a whole new ball game.

The numbers of abandoned children reported for Brazil in 1983 were not totally without historical precedent. During the civil war that devastated the Soviet Union in the 1920s, estimates of the number of abandoned children ("bezprizorniye," literally "without looking after" as they are called in Russian) reached nine million according to Geiger's account in his history of *The Soviet Family*. The fact that Brazil was experiencing such widespread abandonment of children testifies to the civil war–like nature of its economic situation in the 1970s and 1980s. Except in rare cases of psychological or moral dysfunction, parents must be under astounding stress before they will give up their children. The available evidence told us that it was economic and social stress, often in combination with individual family problems, not simple psychopathology or moral breakdown, that was at the root of the problem in Brazil. It was in this sense "structural" rather than "personal".

A major reason for abandoned kids was utter destitution in families that simply could not care for older children once the next wave of infants and toddlers was born. But there was more. The poverty and the vast gap between rich and poor (the sense of relative economic deprivation) in Brazil and other parts of Latin America (and Africa for that matter) was so intense and pervasive it put so much psychological weight on families that many cracked under the pressure. The Gini Index referred to earlier was 59 in Brazil in 1979 and by 1989 it stood at 63—and stood at 57 in 2005. In other words, from the standpoint of income inequality, things in Brazil got worse during the 1980s, and now (after political changes that brought to power a government with its avowed mission being to address the unmet needs of the poor) have returned to where things stood in the 1970s. In 1983, about one third of the households in Brazil had less than one minimum wage, about U.S. $40 per month (at the black market exchange rate current when I visited). The Brazilian state of Rio Grande do Sul used to be so poor, as the saying goes, "If you found a snake you couldn't find a piece of wood to hit it with."

What did the young refugees of Brazil's economic civil war do to survive? They did what young victims of economic disruption have always done. They work when they can, and beg, steal, and sell themselves when they must. They survive or they die. Many die. Most survive. Some even find a way out of their socioeconomic purgatory and into the modern economy located in and around the cities. I saw some of these children during my visit. During the day they were to be seen hustling on the streets—for example, selling sticks of gum or small packets of nuts—or begging. At night they were like ghosts, often sleeping in small groups, huddled together in doorways, parks, or anywhere else they could find (and not be found by the police, who often routed, harassed, and assaulted them). I took pictures that hang on my office wall. Seeing them in person made the heart heavy.

Walking the streets of Brazil's three largest cities, Sao Paulo, Rio, and Belo Horizonte in 1983, I was struck by their Dickensian character. Rio had a special charm, of course, because of its exquisite natural beauty, with its green hills, white beaches, and blue ocean. It was easy to believe at times that Rio was at economic peace, particularly if one stuck to the tourist areas. Viewed from afar, even the shanty towns ("favelas") that climbed the hills and had few if any basic services such as sanitation, running water, and electricity could look picturesque from the tourist's vantage point. But Sao Paulo and Belo did not hide the economic battleground as well as Rio did.

These cities evoked Dickens' London to be sure. Like the London of Dickens' time, the big cities of Brazil offered unmatched splendor for the rich few and appalling squalor for the many poor. For example, I've never had better sushi than in Sao Paulo— and never seen more desperate poverty than I did there. One knew that Fagin, the Artful Dodger, Bill Sikes, Nancy, and Oliver Twist were all there in the back alleys during the day and the main streets at night.

Referring to thievery by kids as the "informal income redistribution system" was a fitting label in a country with little or no public welfare system or safety net. The juvenile detention system—"The Foundation for the Well-Being of Minors"— seemed right out of Dickens' "Nicholas Nickelby" (as film maker Hector Babenco documented in "Pixote," his filmed account of a poor youngster caught up in that system).

There was general agreement among informed observers in Brazil that the problem of abandoned children and youth grew directly in proportion to the "progress" of the economic miracle of export-oriented industrialization in the 1970s. During this time, the impoverished rural areas languished, while the cities became magnets of supposed (and real) opportunity. By 1983, the economic situation had become a kind of Catch-22 double bind for too many of Brazil's children and youth. When economic conditions got worse, children suffered because there was still more unemployment and even less money for basic services. When economic conditions improved, children and youth suffered because the cities became even more powerful magnets, drawing economic refugees from the rural areas and from the chronically impoverished Northeast, with the result being still further crowding and deterioration of urban conditions—more and worse favelas.

When I was there in 1983, an upsurge of street crime attributable to youthful offenders was underway, with a 30% increase from 1982 to 1983, according to one report. Many believed there was a direct correlation between the rate of juvenile crime and the number of abandoned children. Certainly it was hard to imagine a group at greater risk for becoming juvenile criminals than abandoned children and youth. Whether it was on the streets of Rio de Janeiro or New York City, the connection is clear. Geiger described the abandoned children and youth of the Soviet Union in the 1920s in words that describe their Brazilian (and American) counterparts equally well: "Not only did the homeless children present a pitiful spectacle, become diseased and die, but they gradually became a public menace, roaming the streets in gangs and committing every crime and violent act." It is sad that these same words and conditions for children keep repeating over the decades and across continents.

In the Soviet Union, they found that only a comprehensive program of treatment and re-socialization could tame these kids and turn them into socially responsible citizens. It took the collectivist approach of educator-psychologist A. S. Makarenko to accomplish that goal in the Soviet Union in the 1920s and 1930s, and even then it required a society committed to mass mobilization for social change to provide the necessary context (and included the ugly use of penal institutions and even executions for the kids who did not respond to treatment).

Brazil in 1983 offered no such mass mobilization, only occasional isolated successes such as the town of Ipameri, where we visited an effort led by community organizer Margarida Fernandes Horlybon. She found homes, work, and basic education for hundreds of children "in the situation of abandonment."

One of the principal threats posed to human development by severe poverty and income inequality is a kind of moral degradation for everyone, poor and rich, and Brazil presented abundant evidence of this. One day after a morning visit to a desperately poor favela in the city of Juiz de Fora my companions and I were scheduled for lunch at a posh country club, as guests of our institutional host.

As we arrived and perceived the despicable contrast between the magnificent meal before us and the deprivation behind us, my eyes found those of a woman whose face mirrored the moral pain I was feeling. She, the ex-nun, and I, who had once considered joining the clergy, shared one thought: "We must atone for this sin we are about to commit." Wasn't it Sophie Tucker who said, "I've been rich and I've been poor, but rich is better." And guiltier perhaps. But guilt can be either paralyzing or motivating. It can lead to acts of conscience and atonement or denial and repression.

Since 1983, the problems of violence have escalated, as the 2003 film "City of God" makes clear. But what sticks with me from Brazil is a lesson about the significance of protecting the human rights of children. The lesson is this: The physical survival of children reflects the degree to which the infrastructure of a society is in working order. Is there drinkable water? Is there sewage treatment? Is there enough food for little bodies to grow? Are parents available to provide the essential emotional nuts and bolts for a young developing child?

The grossest good measure of all this is the infant mortality rate, the answer to the question, "How many babies die in the first year of life?" There are many amplifications of this number, of course, for example, the child mortality rate after age one and before age five, the rate of environmentally induced mental retardation, the growth and height curves of the children. But the underlying reality of the matter is that if the basic human rights to physical and social care institutions are functioning, parents will care for children, and children will survive. And if they survive—and not seriously malnourished, drastically neglected, or chronically sick—children will smile. It is good to be alive, even if your playground is a garbage dump, even if your toys are pieces of junk, even if your food is boring and tasteless. Children can thrive so long as there is an intact structure of adult support and caring—families with the resources to provide basic care, elementary schools to provide basic education, and some sort of health care system to keep children alive and reasonably free from disease.

However, the criteria for evaluating the human rights of children change with the onset of adolescence. If children are barometers of the physical functioning of their society, then adolescents are social and cultural weathervanes. In their faces and behavior are seen the well-being of the culture and the social structures of the community, and indeed of the whole society. This is the lesson I saw in the faces of the kids I met in Brazil: The children smile, the teenagers frown.

Except for the children who were sick and malnourished, youngsters smile. But even if they are not sick and malnourished, teenagers need more to have a sense of well-being. As they become old enough to envision themselves in the future they need hope and "future orientation." As they become old enough to understand their place in society, they need self-esteem and recognition that their society values them and will make room for them in meaningful ways. As they reach adolescence, they reflect back at us how well the society is doing in creating a sense of deep value and meaningfulness to life, and particularly their lives, as they emerge from childhood and contemplate adulthood. They then begin to participate fully in the moral dilemmas of socioeconomic inequality. They then begin to evidence the corrosive moral effects of poverty—and what it motivates a kid to do or not do.

Or a parent. While visiting a health clinic in a poor section of Sao Paulo in 1983, I was approached by a mother who had her 8-year old daughter in tow. I had noticed her watching me and my group of American professionals for the hour we had been touring the clinic and listening to the director explain their goals, accomplishments, and frustrations. As the rest of the group moved on to see the emergency room I lingered in the pediatrics section, as I often do on such visits. One of our group's translators remained with me as I asked the nurses and the children more questions—and brought out the hand puppets I always take with me on such trips. They never fail to produce smiles and delight among the children, and bringing them out is one the high points of any visit I make to the dark side of human experience.

As I was packing up my puppets to move on, the woman who had been watching me approached, and asked the translator to join us. She said something in Portuguese to the translator, who looked dubious but then resignedly nodded her head. She turned to me and said in English, "This woman has a question for you." "What is it?" I asked. The translator spoke to the woman again in Portuguese. Her answer left the translator shaking her head and visibly upset. "What is it?" I asked again. "She says she wants you to take her daughter—her name is Anna—with you to America so she can have a life. Two of her other children have died of some sickness, and she does not want to lose this one. She says, please take her and give her a life."

With that the woman took the little girl and put her hand in mine. I held it for a time. Then I had to rejoin my group. I left the child behind, and gave her mother some money and my weak apologies. Poverty is about not being regular. It is about your parent being so desperate that she could give you away to save your life. And it is about being left behind. Even more than 20 years later as I recall her pain and the shame of her situation I am angry and sad that this mother and her child and the millions like her must live with the heavy weight of not being "regular." I cried then, and I cry now just remembering it.

My second trip to Brazil took place a quarter of a century later. Since my first trip to Brazil in 1983, political and economic conditions have waxed and waned. Eventually the military dictatorship gave way to a fledgling democracy. In 2002, Luiz Inacio Lula da Silva was elected president, a leader with roots in and commitments to the poor of his country. Time will tell if he can make a difference in the lives of the millions of children whose lives are forfeit without a different way of making economic decisions, but at least this leader has sought to confront the economic realities of Brazil with a commitment to the human rights of poor children.

Da Silva inherited a declining infant mortality rate (from 38 per 1,000 in 2000 to 36 per 1,000 in 2002), and the rate has continued to decline since his administration took office (reaching 28 per 1,000 in 2007, presumably as a reflection of his government's investments in protecting the basic human rights of parents and children in poor families). Time will tell if the commitments made will be fulfilled and the human rights of children protected. But I will say that during my second trip to Brazil no mothers offered their children to me.

Chapter 7
The Right to Equality: No Girl Left Behind

> *When men are oppressed, it's a tragedy. When women are oppressed, it's a tradition.*
>
> —Seen on a bumper sticker

Human rights' advocates have long struggled with the fundamental question of whether or not to focus on subgroups of the human community—for example, the rights of people with disabilities, the elderly, indigenous peoples, and of course, closest to our concern, children. Most clearly resolved of these struggles has been the need to pay special attention to the rights of female human beings—as exemplified in the U.N.'s Declaration of the Elimination of Discrimination Against Women, passed in 1967.

Females stand in the odd position of potentially constituting a majority of the human population by virtue of the many ways in which they are biologically superior (in the sense of being genetically predisposed to longer life expectancy than males), but nonetheless on a global basis of being a subordinate group, with less power, less access to resources, and more victimization than males. For example, the World Health Organization's 2002 *World Report on Violence and Health* reports that "In 48 population-based surveys from around the world, 10–69% of women reported being physically assaulted by an intimate male partner at some point in their lives" (p. 15). A study by the World Bank estimates that in industrialized countries sexual assault and violence take away almost 1 in 5 healthy years of life for women aged 15–44.

The various agencies of the United Nations have documented the inferior status of females around the world—with the exception of a relatively few truly egalitarian societies, such as those in Scandinavia. And these same reports conclude that it is precisely the inequality of women that is linked to the disproportionate rates at which they are victimized. Quoting again from the 2002 WHO report:

> Women are particularly vulnerable to abuse by their partners in societies where there are marked inequalities between men and women, rigid gender roles, cultural norms that support a man's right to sex regardless of a woman's feelings, and weak sanctions against such behavior." (p. 16)

When it comes to female children, issues of inequality are equally pernicious if not more so. This is true across the board, be it access to education (globally, girls are two times more likely to be without education than boys—200 million to 100 million) or selective abortion, infanticide, or neglect (globally, some 60 million girls are "missing" from the population due to gender bias in parental decision making), or involuntary involvement in the sex trade (globally, about 90% of the children sacrificed each year are girls). In almost every domain of the human rights of children, girls are disproportionately unprotected.

Advocates have long struggled with the challenge of finding ways to approach the enormous variations in the severity of human rights issues across the range of societies in the world. On the one hand, there are the gross human rights abuses of girls in the most patriarchal and sexually oppressive societies, where the issues of survival, illiteracy, and sexual exploitation dominate. On the other, there are the more subtle but nonetheless psychologically significant issues faced by girls in the societies in which gender egalitarianism has made progress, issues such as persistent disparities in earnings and disproportionate rates of non-lethal victimization.

Most child advocates resist a moral calculus that dismisses the significance of the latter class of issues because of its relatively smaller impact on suffering and deprivation (what is often called the "classification of oppression"). *All* suffering merits our concern; *all* human rights violations demand redress. This is the only way to hold in one's heart and mind the two ends of the severity spectrum of oppression—from the widespread brutalization of girls in the Thai sex trade to the objectification of American girls on television. But there is no denying that the abuses at the most severe end must have a distinctive moral claim on our resources and attention, and we will return to the most severe end of that spectrum later. First let's consider how the human rights of girls are violated in a relatively progressive society such as the United States.

When the great American anthropologist Margaret Mead was pregnant, she and her husband Gregory Bateson debated where to raise their child. According to her autobiography, *Blackberry Winter*, Mead tells us that the couple decided that if the baby was a boy they should live in England, but if the baby was a girl they should live in the United States. Why? Both of them believed America was a less sexist, less patriarchal world than England, and a girl in the United States would have a better chance of growing up without feeling like she was a second-class citizen. Their daughter Mary Catherine Bateson was born in 1939, they raised her in the United States, and she grew up to be a very modern woman.

Of course even in the United States with its constitutional rhetoric of freedom, attaining equality of females has been a long time coming (and is not yet fully realized). In many concrete ways, females were second-class citizens from the start, as evidenced by the fact that it was not until 1920, with passage of the nineteenth amendment to the Constitution and extension of voting rights to women, did females achieve even a modicum of political equality as citizens. The gender inequalities and political agitation that led to passage of the amendment did not stop with gaining the right to vote, of course. Both continued through the 1930s, and it was not until the latter part of the twentieth century that gender equality began to really take hold in the United States.

For example, it wasn't until the 1970s that law and legal practice began to revoke the "right" of a man to beat his wife that many men seemed to believe came with a marriage license—which is not to say that wife beating has stopped by any means in the United States. Viewed from a universal egalitarian perspective on human rights, America has not achieved full equity between men and women, but we have come a long way. Both in comparison with where we started and in contrast with many other societies even today, American women are liberated. But what has all this social change meant for girls? In one sense that's an easy question to answer: The result has been the unleashing of girls from the oppression of the patriarchal values and social structures and the corresponding blossoming of opportunities for all kids.

Equality is good for girls for many reasons, including basic developmental processes. As psychologist Emmy Werner has found around the world, research on resilience reveals that traditional girls who have only "feminine" characteristics are at a disadvantage (as are traditionally sex-typed boys, for that matter). They are less flexible and less likely to access social resources that can increase power to master the challenges the world may present. In contrast, the most resilient girls are those who combine in their repertoire of characteristics such traditionally masculine traits as being autonomous and independent (rather than being passive and dependent) with their traditionally feminine traits, such as emotional expressivity, social perceptiveness, and nurturance.

The term androgyny refers to this human completeness. Put simply, androgyny enhances resilience. The same goes for boys, by the way. It's akin to saying that kids are more adaptable when they have both hands free than when they have one hand tied behind their backs, even if they are right- or left-handed.

How does androgyny arise developmentally? It flows from two basic changes, one cultural, the other social. The cultural change flows from altering the messages sent to girls by adults—directly as parents and teachers, and indirectly via the mass media and other public institution. Every time girls receive the message that "good girls don't do X" in a situation in which boys *can* do X, the foundation for androgyny suffers. Egalitarian messages build this foundation. Thus, shifting the cultural messages changes the definition of what is possible and legitimate for girls. In Chapter 4 I introduced the concept of "cognitive structuring." Here it is a useful term to use in understanding how the idea of what a girl is and is entitled to changes as culture and society change.

The social dimension of this change lies in opening the full range of developmentally enhancing experiences to girls. By being allowed into new settings—such as competitive sports, for example—or better still, being invited and welcomed, girls get to experience "behavioral rehearsal" of new skills and attitudes. The combination of cognitive structuring and behaviorally rehearsing egalitarianism enhances the androgyny and thus the resilience of girls. And in the United States, progress toward androgyny for girls is evident in the way superior functioning of girls is increasing—for example, graduating from high school and entering college at higher rates, earning more than males during the first two decades of adult life, and in other ways improving the lot of girls as egalitarianism and thus androgyny increases for females (probably more so than for males).

However, there is more to this matter of the basic human rights of girls than protection from assault, neglect, and social deprivation, on the one hand, and opening up previously closed behavioral settings on the other. One of the underlying issues is the matter of acceptance versus rejection. Human beings have evolved to thrive in conditions in which they are accepted and languish when they are rejected. This is one of the few "universals" in child development. Rejection is about actions that send the message "You are not good enough," and thus offer a negative definition of self to a child. As anthropologist Ronald Rohner documented in his 1975 book, *They Love Me, They Love Me Not*, and in hundreds of studies since then, rejection is universally a psychological malignancy, an emotional cancer that disrupts development and distorts behavior.

This is relevant to our concern with the human rights of girls because one way to understand the global situation of girls is to see the pervasive messages of rejection that are embedded in the sexist world order. Over and over again, and with increasing severity as we move along the continuum from progressive-egalitarian societies at one end of the spectrum, to oppressive-patriarchal societies at the other end, we can see escalating messages of rejection being directed at girls. These are the messages that say "because you are a girl you are not good enough to be educated, you are not good enough to be in control of your sexual integrity and privacy, you are not good enough to vote, you are not good enough to earn as much as boys, you are not good enough to play with boys, you are not good enough to be fed as much as boys, you are not good enough to pray with boys," and so on and so on. It is all about messages of rejection, rejection just because you are a girl.

This, I think, is what links together the grotesque violations of rape and abuse with the more subtle violations of oppressive sexism and patriarchy. They both contain messages of rejection and are thus psychologically damaging. This is where the human rights issue starts, with the psychological violence done to girls that establishes the foundation for all the other violence and neglect they disproportionately experience in the world, at home and abroad. For me, all this came to a head on a visit to Sudan in 1985.

Case Study: Protecting Girls in Sudan

Sudan is a country of about 40 million people located in Northeast Africa, just south of Egypt. A former British colony (when it was called "The Sudan"), it is a harsh and poor land through which the Nile River flows. Until oil reserves were discovered in the latter part of the twentieth century it had few prospects for wealth. Its capital is Khartoum, the site of a famous battle in 1882 between the British Army under General Gordon and the Muslim forces of the Mahdi, and site of the 2002 movie "The Four Feathers." When I was preparing for my trip in 1985, a military government with strong Islamic fundamentalist inclinations was in power, having overthrown the old corrupt civilian government of President Nimeiri just before my visit.

Few Americans go to Sudan. Rarely does it figure in the news. Exceptions include the U.S. 1997 bombing of buildings suspected to be making weapons for Osama Bin Laden's Al Qaeda terrorists, an occasional story about the civil war pitting the Muslim government in the north against the Christian and "Animist" people of the south, and now the ongoing awfulness of the ethnic cleansing and genocide in the Darfur region. Also, there are periodic feature stories about "The Lost Boys of Sudan," chronicling the bands of abandoned and orphaned kids who roamed Sudan and nearby countries looking for sanctuary, some of whom were eventually repatriated to the United States. I went to Sudan in 1985 to visit two children— Shama and Hamad—who my family and I had been supporting through a private international charity originally called the International Foster Parent Plan (and at that time redefining itself as PLAN International).

My visit to Hamad was moving in many respects. As my PLAN International translator and I approached his family's walled compound I saw Hamad. The black and white pictures we received from PLAN were clear enough for me to be pretty sure it was he. He was smiling and looked a bit ragged. His mother and baby brother were there too; his father was working somewhere away from the village hauling water. Hamad's family house had one room, about 15′ × 15′, and a couple of beds and a table with the pots and dishes. I gave him the gifts I had brought from home—a stuffed animal (a lion) and a baseball cap from Penn State University (where I was teaching at the time). He beamed shyly and held onto the lion while I took his picture. I enjoyed my time with this little boy.

I was introduced to his mother (and grandmother and two aunts) and then all that I had heard about the cultural issues involved in the concept of "foster parent plan" for Sudan came to life. Hamad's mother feared I had come to claim her son. A belief which eventually gave way to the reassurance I offered through the translator. The mother had two other sons, both of whom had died (not statistically surprising in a country with 50% mortality among children by 5 and another 10% from then until age 10, but horrifying nonetheless). Hamad's community was particularly old-fashioned, which in Sudanese society translates into immunization rates of 5%, zero family planning, and the fact that every single mother in the community has had at least one child die—every single one! It's a sobering reminder of what extreme poverty is about.

But the most disturbing element of this visit was not my time spent with Hamad. It was my visit with Shama, our other sponsored child. Why? Because meeting Shama put a human face to the practice of genital mutilation, and provided a vivid demonstration of why any concern for the human rights of children must have a special focus on the human rights of girls.

Before coming to Sudan in 1985, I had read about female genital mutilation, but had not yet confronted it directly. From what I had read I knew enough to be outraged, but still found it hard to stomach the fact that all the girls in a community like Shama's would have their exterior genitalia cut off—often with no anesthesia and with lousy sanitary conditions—and have their vaginal opening sown up to the size of a pin hole.

There has been a lot of academic discussion of this issue in Europe and North America as an abstract consideration of culture and patriarchy, but there it was in front of me. As I walked through Shama's village on the way to her house I could not shake the thought that *all* of these young girls had been mutilated. Meeting her big complex family—aunts, grandmother, mother—I could not shake the thought, because I knew that the physical consequences of this mutilation include the retention of urine and menstrual blood, infections, sometimes sterility, frequent problems with childbirth, and always destruction of the capacity for sexual gratification (because the clitoris is the primary target of the procedure). It is horrible, however culturally normal it is here. Not just non-Sudanese recognize this—to wit a book by a Sudanese female physician Dr. Asma el Dareer entitled, *Women Why Do You Weep*?

At age eight, Shama was right at the age when the horror was most likely to be done to her. Shama was as she appeared in the PLAN photo I carried, although prettier it seemed to me. She was quite shy, and reluctant at first to sit with me, so the translator sat next to her and everyone crowded into the little house. But there was none of the fear of me kidnapping her that Hamad and his family evidenced, just good old-fashioned shyness. The little girl was very slender and dressed in a green, Western-style dress for the big occasion of my visit.

There were several little girls hanging around the courtyard outside Shama's little house. All clad in Western dresses, the girls were between 5 and 15 years of age, and very much looked to one of the grandmothers present for direction—she was obviously the matriarch of this extended family compound. In the corner of the one room in Shama's home there was a wooden cabinet with glass doors, the site of the family's treasures: pots, pans, a few china pieces, and some glasses. Stuck to the doors were the pictures of me and my family. I passed around the current pictures of my son Josh and daughter Joanna that I had brought with me, and they were kept as souvenirs of my visit.

The PLAN translator was intent on pushing Shama toward me. Her reluctance was clear, so I tried to direct everyone's attention elsewhere. The translator and her mother ordered her to hug me. Much as I would have liked to have a hug, I knew it is ludicrous to demand it of the shy little girl. I was a very foreign stranger to her, despite the fact there was a picture of me in the china cabinet. So I did what I always do, I pulled out my puppets.

Shama was afraid at first, but her infant baby brother smiled and reached out for them. So he got to look at them until Shama had enough time to warm up to me. And then she accepted graciously the toy lion I had brought with me, smiled her lovely shy smile, and even accepted the required hug.

Before we left her house I was offered a drink—in a glass on a special tray set on the one table in the house. My hesitation was only momentary, but the grandmother noticed and demanded that I drink it. Courtesy is more powerful than gastrointestinal self-interest, so I complied as best I could—leaving as much in the glass as I thought was within the limits of politeness. We drove off and I had one final look at these lovely girls and women. But my vision of them was clouded by the nagging knowledge that each of them has been genitally mutilated—even precious little Shama.

At a later point in my trip I broached the subject of female genital mutilation with PLAN's Sudan program director. He cited the usual facts: It was nearly 100% prevalent in the rural areas, it was a Sudanese, not a Muslim tradition (although often presented as Muslim), and PLAN could not say a word about it in public.

He did tell me a story, however: A European-educated Sudanese man he knew forbade the mutilation of his two daughters, aged 9 and 11. When the man was away for 2 weeks attending a professional conference in Europe, his wife gave in to the pressure of the two grandmothers to have the girls cut. When he returned home to discover what had happened he was enraged but could do nothing. He walked out in despair and got drunk with a friend, only later that night to be informed that the younger girl, age 9, had died from an infection. He was so angry with his wife that he had not spoken to her in the last 2 years. An important point for future thought: The custom is driven by the vicious patriarchy but implemented by the women.

But the positive potential of this horrible story reminds me of how foot binding was challenged and stopped in China. Progress really began when progressive men started declaring in public that they would not marry any girl with bound feet, this as a way to support the movement against foot binding. I suspect it will take something like that here to make significant progress toward ending this abomination. I hate to think of little Shama being mutilated. As a father myself with a beloved daughter it shocks and disturbs me to the core.

The PLAN Director told me that some of the beggars I have seen on the streets of Khartoum are handless because of the application of strict Sharia (Islamic law) that calls for chopping off the hands of thieves. It is part of the fundamentalist agenda, which includes attacks on women for offenses such as showing their ankles. He reports that some Western women have been stoned in villages because they were "immodestly dressed."

So many of the women here are locked into that conservative system—in part, I think, because "misery loves company"—but mostly because they have so little that they have to protect what little they have in a nasty social order. They are trapped and demand that every other woman and girl be trapped too. And some, of course, seek to protect girls from danger by identifying them as within the party line—genital mutilation being the most vivid example.

Un-mutilated girls are the target of peer pressure; for example, they are labeled "loose." Their parents are warned, "You'll be sorry when she is loose and wanton." It's quite an interlocking system. Men say it is a feminine matter, but make it clear that they support it. Women say they do it for the men, but reinforce it by more than passive acceptance. Will it change? I don't know. (But now 20 years later I know that it has continued.)

I find it virtually impossible to adopt a position of "cultural relativism" on the matter of female genital mutilation when I think of dear little Shama. Sure, there are terrible things that happen in my own country—abuse and neglect—and much of my professional life has been devoted to seeking remedies. But what about when I leave my home country and culture and travel to a place and society that is as foreign to me as Sudan?

A friend of mine who teaches Islamic law reports that in teaching undergraduates to suspend their Western biases he asks them to consider the relative horror of the traditional Islamic punishment for theft—chopping off a hand—and the American practice of putting the offender in prison for a period of years during which time they are likely to be brutalized sexually and emotionally and emerge with a self-defeating and socially destructive negative attitude. Food for thought, thought about the magnitude and diversity of human rights abuses in the world.

I agree totally that the cultural traveler must be careful and self-aware to the highest possible level and with greatest possible soul-searching before judging another culture. But I cannot shake the belief that there is something different about the routine genital mutilation of girls in Sudan and other countries in Africa and elsewhere. The idea that all cultural practices are equivalent and cannot be judged by other cultures seems impossible to sustain in this case. In fact, this example gives rise to an enduring theme in my writing and lecturing about the role of cultural differences in human development.

I think it is crucial to the enterprise of advancing human development to recognize that not all cultural differences are the same and equal. Some differences surely are only matters of style; for example, whether you keep your hat on or take it off when entering a place of worship. Others reflect the pursuit of different goals for socialization; for example, the Hawaiian interest in producing cooperative, group-oriented people in contrast to the goal of producing rugged individualists in North America.

But surely there is a third kind of cultural difference, when the culture is "wrong." This may be because the practice is obsolete in light of changed circumstances (and thus may become harmful since its original justification is no longer valid). It may be because it is inconsistent with the fundamental values and principles of the society (a kind of mistake that can be rectified by pointing out the inconsistency). It may be "wrong" because it rests upon a factually incorrect belief (such as the idea that children develop best when they are exposed to chronic shame and humiliation leading to a feeling of rejection). It may be because it violates the universal standards of human rights that flow from each child being God's child. All these are sources of "wrongness" in cultural practices regarding the treatment of children.

Swiss psychoanalyst Alice Miller has offered us a concept that captures this idea well. She calls it "poisonous pedagogy" (using pedagogy in the European sense of "upbringing" or "socialization" as opposed to the typical American usage as "teaching"). By poisonous pedagogy she means practices that are normal but wrong, normal in the sense of being culturally approved and statistically common, wrong in the sense of being misguided as to their developmental impact and their violating universal human good—messing with God's children, if you will.

Naturally, it is easier to recognize poisonous pedagogy in a foreign culture in which one does not have a personal stake than it is in one's home society—where the need to protectively rationalize and justify harmful practices is great. This is one reason why we need international efforts like the U.N. Convention on the Rights of the Child, to help each society and culture to take an "objective" look at what otherwise seems obvious and a given.

Though not ratified in 1985 when I was in Sudan (that came in 1991), the U.N. Convention on the Rights of the Child has come to symbolize for me this last matter: a universal statement of the basics of human rights for children and a universal definition of what it should mean to be a child. The genital mutilation of girls in Sudan is surely a violation, something so clearly wrong it turns my stomach and weighs on my heart no matter how informed I become of its cultural significance and history. It is gratifying to see that some Sudanese can themselves see it.

The global community has been involved in a long period of waking up to the fact that the oppression of girls (and women) is the driving force behind much of the worst suffering in the world—from gang rape as a terrorist tactic in Darfur and the former Yugoslavia, to the genital mutilation and educational deprivation of girls in Africa, to the fact that domestic violence is virulent as a direct function of the patriarchal oppression of women throughout the world.

I look through the eyes of the U.N. Convention on the Rights of the Child and see my own culture and society better and with greater insight because I have traveled to other cultures and societies (and grieve the fact that my government has still not ratified it). The Convention is a shining piece of evidence that there can be a way to walk the line between passive acceptance of violations of children in the name of "cultural relativism" and wrong-headed imposition of one culture's standards upon another through military or economic force in the name of cultural imperialism. Here the force is more sublime; it is the force of looking at suffering directly and seeing it for what it is and who it serves. This, for me, was the lesson of Sudan, the lesson taught to me by the suffering of these girls in a very extreme situation. We must anchor our analyses of children's lives with the concept of human rights applied judiciously, respectfully, and with humility, but applied nonetheless, particularly when it comes to the oppression of the female children of the world.

Chapter 8
Home and Homeland: Displaced Children and Youth

Home is the place where

when you have to go there

they have to take you in.

—Robert Frost

Children have a right to be at home and to have a homeland. This right flows from their need to be anchored somewhere psychologically, to be part of something stable and enduring, something larger than themselves where they can feel a non-contingent sense of belonging. When this right is violated and this need unmet, children are adrift, and in being adrift they are candidates for losing their way in the world.

Children live in and through their "social maps." Each such map is both the product of past experience and the cause of future actions. Some children see themselves as powerful, secure countries, surrounded by allies. Others see themselves as poor little islands, surrounded by an empty ocean or hostile enemies.

Such representations of the world reflect a child's intellectual ability—the cognitive competence of knowing the world in an objective sense—but they also indicate moral and emotional inclinations. Children develop social maps, and then they live by them—as we saw in Chapter 4, where we looked at how the social maps of abused children can put them on the fast track to conduct disorder. In early childhood, the outlines of these social maps begin to emerge. What we commonly call "attachment" is the first such map. It reflects the way an infant understands the social environment. Some infants have a strong, positive map of attachment, and live a life of responsiveness and security. For them the social map of attachment provides a foundation for exploration—physically and emotionally—because it provides a secure base of human operations, a secure mini-homeland.

Without this starting point in positive attachment, however, the human child is psychologically homeless, and the social map begins to emerge without appropriate boundaries, allies, and orientation to emotional north, south, east, and west. Cultures differ in the precise components of these early social maps, of course. For example, in some societies, fathers provide intimate care for infants and emerge in their attachment maps early on, whereas in other societies fathers do not appear in childhood social maps until later on, but the universal truth is that someone must be "on the map."

J. Garbarino, *Children and the Dark Side of Human Experience.*
© Springer Science+Business Media, LLC 2008

The psychoanalyst Erik Erikson proposed that children must find their way through a series of major challenges en route to a healthy adulthood. These "crises" require that the child construct a social map that will show the way. The first potential roadblock is "basic trust versus distrust." Does the child come to know the world as a reliable place, where needs are met (basic trust), or as a chaotic place where needs go unmet (basic distrust)?

If children can navigate through this challenge, they continue down the road of positive development. Other potential roadblocks lie ahead, such as failing to become competent in dealing with bodily issues like toilet training as a toddler, failing to develop a balanced approach to adult authority as a school-aged child, and failing to develop a solid positive identity as an adolescent.

The social map continues to develop in ways that reflect the child's experiences and emerging capacities. What's more, the social map more and more becomes the cause of experience. By adolescence, a youth is always acting upon the basis of the information within the map. The youth whose map contains allies acts confidently and securely, and increasingly finds the positive places in life. The youth whose map renders him or her an insignificant speck stuck off in a corner accrues more and more negative experiences. Not surprisingly, research reveals that troubled and delinquent youth are disproportionately likely to have disrupted attachment relationships.

We are concerned with the conclusions about the world contained in a child's social map. Will it be "I belong here," "Adults are to be trusted because they know what they are doing," "People will generally treat you well and meet your needs," "I am a valued member of my society," and "The future looks bright to me"? Or will it be "I have no place to call home," "Strangers are dangerous," "School is a dangerous place," "I feel all alone," and "All I see in my future is more disappointment and failure"?

Just what are the boundaries of a child's social map, a child's home? The great spiritual teachers from all the world's faith traditions teach us that the boundaries are not limited to the material and observable world. They extend outward to the universe and inward to the soul. But how are we to study and understand these non-material dimensions of being at home?

H.L. Mencken offered an introduction to the concept of home when he wrote:

> A home is not a mere transient shelter. Its essence lies in its permanence, in its capacity for accretion and solidification, in its quality of representing, in all its details, and the personalities of the people who live in it.

The focal point of both the quote from Robert Frost's poem "Death of the Handyman" that began this chapter and Mencken's observations is that "home" implies permanence and stability. You have a home when you have a place to go, no matter what. You have a home when you are connected permanently with a place that endures and represents your family. As a young homeless child wrote, "A home is where you can grow flowers if you want."

It's only a small step from this concept of home to the political idea of homeland as a sense that you are part of a nation, that you belong somewhere politically.

Children and youth around the world are often caught up in adult struggles to define and defend homeland—or in the case of some displaced groups—to re-establish or create a homeland (as has long been the case for groups such as the Kurds, Tamils, Palestinians, Zionist Jews prior to the creation of the modern state of Israel, and many indigenous peoples around the world).

I have had a chance to witness the importance of identity and the ways in which political forces can distort the natural process of identity formation for kids when concepts of identity and homeland are in crisis. I saw this acutely in Croatia during the war that followed upon the breakup of the former Yugoslavia in the 1990s. Kids need a positive identity: You have to be someone, preferably someone positive, and having a place to call home is part of that process. I learned this lesson anew because of the day I sat in a refugee camp school near Zagreb with a group of eight kids ranging in age from 11 to 13.

All these kids had suffered from the war. Thirteen-year-old Adriana was a refugee from Sarajevo who simply sat and cried when asked about the future. Thirteen-year-old Petra came from a nearby village, but was displaced to Zagreb when his house was burned in a raid by Serbian forces—some of whom used to be his neighbors. Before he escaped to the capital city of Zagreb with his mother, 11-year-old Diepo was caught on the front lines, and witnessed the defeat of his father's militia in the battle for their town. Eleven-year-old Klago lived with his family in Sofia (Serbia), but had to leave when the war started because of their Croatian heritage. The list went on as Marco, Christina, and Paula joined the others in telling their tales of woe. Finally, there sat 12-year-old Maria. She lived in Sarajevo but then fled to Dubrovnik and Sofia before ending up here in Zagreb, with her mother and her mother's family—her father left behind somewhere along the way.

After some discussion I asked each child, "What are you?" "Croatian," says Adriana without hesitation. "Croatian," echoes Petra firmly. "Croatian," answers Paula. "Croatian," says Diepo with obvious pride. "Croatian," continues Klajo. "Croatian," concurs Marco. Cristina also has no doubts, "Croatian," she says. Then all eyes turned to Maria. "Yugoslavian," she says, looking directly at me and not at her peers. All seven other pair of eyes turn on her, each face broadcasting a negative message. Distain. Anger. Hostility. Rage. Disappointment. There wasn't a positive face in the room except for me, the professional outsider (and perhaps the translator, although given the situation, I'm not completely sure of her).

"Why on earth is this girl holding onto a Yugoslavian identity when everyone else has 'reverted' to being Croatian?" I wondered. So I asked her about it. "What does it mean to you to be Yugoslavian?" I asked her. "My father is Russian and my mother is Croatian," she replied, "and I am Yugoslavian."

That was it. For her, being Yugoslavian was a solution to her ethnically mixed parentage. For the others, being Croatian was a simple answer for the simple problem of being "not them." Like most of their compatriots, they had never really been Yugoslavian, only Croats in waiting. They had no intrinsic need for Yugoslavia, at least none that they were aware of.

But this little girl had had a very practical need that being Yugoslavian fulfilled. It allowed her to be something without choosing between her parents. The message from her peers was very clear in that schoolroom in Zagreb: "You can no longer be Yugoslavian. You are either with us—Croatian—or against us—Serbian or Bosnian." What a choice for a child—or an adult for that matter—to have to make! Maria was refusing their choice and trying to hold on the best answer for her particular situation.

The U.N. Convention on the Rights of the Child guarantees every child an identity. Article 8 commits governments "to respect the right of the child to preserve his or her identity, including nationality, name and family relations as recognized by law without unlawful interference." Indeed, the Convention is the only U.N. statement on human rights that includes this particular commitment. It's a wise commitment, grounded in developmental theory and research. Every child has to be someone, hopefully someone he or she can be proud of, and having a place to call your own is part of that.

But how does this right to identity mesh with other rights and the developmental needs of children? For example, sometimes the needs of children for quality care may conflict with the right to a cultural identity. Let me cite two situations to illustrate this point. First, when African-American children are abandoned or are removed because of child maltreatment and then are placed with White parents (or vice versa) some advocates have argued that this violates the child's right to cultural identity. Naturally, these advocates acknowledge the child's right to be safe from neglect and abuse, but sometimes seem to put cultural identity ahead of these more standard considerations of the "best interest" of the child.

Second, some Tibetan children (including some close to me personally) have been separated from their parents (with the parents' acquiescence, even enthusiastic endorsement) to attend boarding schools principally as a method of ensuring the continuity of Tibetan cultural identity in exile. Here again the rights of the child to cultural identity and a supportive family life seem to be in conflict. How might we resolve the dilemma of these conflicting rights?

I think the key to resolving this dilemma flows from a developmental perspective. In this case that means recognizing that the needs (and therefore rights) of children may well be different from the needs (and rights) of adolescents. Specifically, what children need is protection, nurturance, love, and day-to-day continuity and quality of care. This is where their "best interest" lies, because their sense of cultural identity (indeed their need for it) is not yet well developed.

In adolescence issues of identity become salient and insistent. Thus, for adolescents, the right to culture is crucially in their best interest. Adolescents who as children are removed from what would ordinarily become their culture may well experience confusion and a sense of loss—most likely, of course, when there are physical correlates of culture that identify the child (most notably in the case of race). However important the needs and rights of adolescents are, though, they should not preempt meeting the developmental needs of *children*. This is particularly important because children who face issues of cultural identity discontinuity in adolescence are almost inevitably facing the personal identity issues that flow from being adopted.

Happily, there is every reason to believe that adolescents who were well cared for as children will have had their basic developmental needs met, and thus will have the psychological and social resources necessary to wrestle effectively with the issue of cultural identity productively (and with the personal identity issues of adoption as well). In contrast, if the child's need for care in the early years is sacrificed on behalf of the need for and right to cultural identity, the result is likely to be disastrous.

Child protection trumps cultural continuity in childhood, and developmentally speaking, a successful childhood is the best predictor of adolescent success (even success in dealing with the feelings of cultural identity crisis that may well come when the well-cared-for child has to deal with cultural disconnection as an adolescent). Of course, the ideal situation is one in which child protection and cultural identity come together easily as a complete and integrated package: biological parents who care for the child and provide cultural continuity for the adolescent.

One aspect of cultural identity is nationality, or as it is more and more likely to be expressed in public discourse today, homeland. Having seen the importance of homeland in times and places of conflict and violence, I wonder what exactly is the meaning of homeland for Americans? I find historian Amy Kaplan's analysis of homeland to be particularly useful. As Kaplan sees it, "homeland connotes an inexorable connection to a place deeply rooted in the past" (p. 84). In World War II the dominant terms was "the home front" (in contrast to the front lines across the oceans, where the fighting was taking place).

It was not a term used during the Cold War either. Kaplan notes that homeland is:

> a term that did not seem historically part of the traditional arsenal of patriotic idiom. Why not domestic security? Civil defense? National security? How many Americans, even at moments of fervent nationalism, think of America as a homeland? How many think of America as their country, nation, home, but think of places elsewhere as their historical ethnic, or spiritual homeland?" (p. 85)

Yet in the view of the *Oxford English Dictionary*, the historical meaning of homeland speaks of "a state, region or territory that is closely identified with a particular people or ethnic group."

Here's what the first head of the Department of Homeland Security had to say about this concept:

> We will work to ensure that the essential liberty of the American people is protected, that terrorists will not take away our way of life. It's called Homeland Security. While the effort will begin here, it will require the involvement of America at every level. Everyone in the homeland must play a part. I ask the American people for their patience, their awareness and their resolve. This job calls for a national effort. We've seen it before, whether it was building the Trans-Continental Railroad, fighting World War II, or putting a man on the moon.

Homeland security is about mobilizing the power of the state and marshaling the efforts of the citizenry.

There are a number of inspiring elements of this message, but there are also some dark shadows that must be confronted. Where do immigrants fit into the homeland? What about people who are citizens but retain a cultural loyalty to another society? What about the ironic position of Native Americans in relation to this homeland? What about people who stand in opposition to the current American regime? These are all important questions, but from the perspective of the right of children to home and homeland these questions are subordinate to a more psychological concern, a concern with identity, with who you are.

I believe that both home and homeland are important in figuring out who you are; that is, in the process of identity formation. Based upon my experience with displaced people around the world, I'm inclined to believe that if you lack either or both (home and homeland) you are likely to suffer from problems of alienation, rootlessness, and depression. This is one way to approach the issue of homeland insecurity, to link it to the way children and youth experience home.

What do we see when we begin this process? We see that there are a lot of children experiencing a sense of insecurity when it comes to home itself. When we look around, we see more and more children and youth growing up with a sense of rootlessness that comes from the experience of family disintegration.

For young children, the concept of home is closely allied with the concept of family. In fact, for very young children, it is hard to separate the two: "My home is where my family lives." Like turtles, young children carry their homes around with them, as they are carried along by their families. This is why when the social environment of parents is disrupted it translates into psychological harm for the children.

Anything that affects the availability of parents and their ability to create and sustain a home for a young child is bad news. Research on children in war zones around the world tells us that young children can cope well with the stress of social upheaval if they retain strong positive attachments to their families, and parents can continue to project a sense of stability, permanence, and competence to their children.

One implication is that when parents of young children have trouble functioning (which may be linked to their sense of being homeless), we can expect negative effects on those children. It is difficult for a family to function well without a home (both in the narrow sense of having a permanent residence and in the larger sense of being part of an intact community).

This is one way to interpret Kai Erikson's study of families who lost their homes and their community as the result of a devastating flood. In his book, *Everything in Its Path*, Erikson highlighted the subsequent difficulties encountered by these families who sought simultaneously to build new homes and a new community. His study directs our attention to the intense social toxicity that arises when whole communities become uprooted. For very young children the principal danger is that a demolished community will demoralize their parents. For older children and adolescents there is another danger, that the lack of community itself will prove harmful. But the story is not simple. These traumatic events can later become the basis for spiritual and psychological growth and development in later life if there is a process of therapeutic recovery.

Once children leave the period of infancy and early childhood (at approximately age 8), their well-being comes to depend more and more upon social realities beyond the immediate family. Their experiences extend in wider circles beyond the family into the neighborhood and community. At the same time, home becomes more than family. It includes school, neighborhood, and friends.

Children appreciate being home in new and different ways as they develop. For a child to have a home is for that child to have a family that lives somewhere, that belongs someplace. A family with a home has a place to call its own (putting aside matters like legal ownership, which are virtually meaningless to a child). Such a family may recognize the possibility of moving in the future to another place, but carries with it the expectation that this new place will become a new home.

Why does the young child equate home and family? It follows from the limited ability of young children to engage in abstract thinking. Young children think in concrete terms, and this concrete thinking makes it likely that "home" and "family" will be the same. What about older children? For them, home and family are separable. A friend of our family announced her intention of moving to a new apartment once her daughter graduated from high school and moved on to college. "But I'll never have a home again," the daughter lamented.

I myself remember my own loss of "home" more than 40 years ago, with the kind of vividness that only emotionally laden memories can sustain. When I was 18 my parents moved from the house in which we had lived since I was 7 years old to a new community 20 miles away. The move took place while I was away at college, so when Thanksgiving break came I traveled to the new house but knew that I could never go home again as a child. I knew that only by getting married and having children of my own could I really have a home again.

My own children felt the same way when we moved from our home in Chicago into a temporary apartment, en route to a permanent move to Ithaca, NY. They had a roof over their heads, yet they felt homeless during the transitional period. I recall with pain suggesting to my 12-year-old daughter Joanna that we "go home" (to the new apartment) and her replying, "I have no home." It took time and experience to make the new house into a home. Her pain flowed from the violation of her right be at home.

"New home" is a shaky concept, a contradiction in terms. This is what my daughter was telling me. For a child to accept a new home is an act of faith. The child is asked to believe that a new place will become a home. A new home is an expectation of stability—a promise, not a fact. It is a commitment to put down roots to build relationships, memories, traditions, associations, and images. This is what it means to tell a child that he or she is home in a new house and neighborhood.

For a child, home is a crucial feature of the social map, and when it is missing, the child may be set adrift and put in jeopardy. This is one important reason why we are concerned about the disruptions of family life that are part of the social toxicity of growing up in America: They are one more challenging to the critical process of forming a stable and positive identity.

Researchers and theoreticians of human development have long emphasized the central importance of identity in adolescence. Erik Erikson went so far as to postulate that forming a stable and positive identity was *the* challenge of adolescence (which if unmet would impede future development in adulthood). Being an immigrant to the United States and thus acutely aware of what it means to be a foreigner, Erikson had a sense that identity had cultural and ethnic dimensions. What is more, he studied Native American kids and cultural icons such as Gandhi and Martin Luther, and was attuned to the importance of who you are as more than an individual matters. Others have refined and improved upon Erikson's approach, but the preoccupation with identity remains a core concern for students of adolescence.

I have seen the way homelessness and being cut off from your homeland affects kids, whether Palestinian kids who live in a perpetual sense of uprootedness because of the loss of their homeland, Vietnamese kids whose status as "boat people" drives them into a similar limbo, or kids in the Balkans struggling with who they are in the wake of the disintegration of Yugoslavia and the resurgence of old nationalist impulses.

The struggle between Israel and the Palestinians provides a poignant illustration of how central homeland is to the social identity of children and youth. At the core of the struggle is a profound disagreement about issues related to homeland and homeland security, a disagreement that has long fueled terrorism. Israel, like the United States, is a nation born of terrorism. Just as American patriots engaged in terrorist actions against the British colonial government in the eighteenth century, Zionist military and paramilitary organizations like the Irgun engaged in terrorist actions against the British colonial administration in the territory of Palestine (and against their Arab rivals for the territory) in the twentieth century. Like terrorists everywhere, they justified their actions as politically necessary and saw themselves as freedom fighters using the traditional tools of the militarily weak, namely, shootings and bombings designed to undermine the morale and will of their enemies through the creation of a state of terror.

Once the State of Israel was declared in 1948, the issues revolved around the efforts of Israel's Arab enemies to disrupt and eventually destroy the Jewish homeland. Those enemies included neighboring Arab states—Jordan, Egypt, Syria, Iraq, and the other countries of the region—as well as Arabs living within Israeli-controlled territories (who increasingly identified themselves as Palestinians and eventually constituted themselves as the Palestine Liberation Organization to coordinate their struggle).

Homeland is certainly a dominant theme in Palestinian culture, perhaps as much as it is in Israel. Homeland is what drives the struggle in the region. The core dispute is precisely the question of whether the territory is the Israeli or Palestinian homeland.

From the perspective of a neutral observer (a hard thing to be in this conflict) both sides make a compelling case for their ancestral right to the land east of the Mediterranean Sea between Lebanon to the north and Egypt to the south extending at least to the city of Jerusalem and perhaps beyond to the Jordan River—the biblical lands of Judea and Sumaria (today often referred to as The West Bank). Most unbiased observers believe that the basis for an eventual political solution will be an Israeli state that ends at Jerusalem and a Palestinian state that begins there and continues to the Jordan River with the addition of the tiny parcel of land to the south of Israel known as the Gaza Strip.

Of course, anyone with a little historical knowledge and a sense of irony is quick to recognize the parallels in the decades of desire to create the Palestinian homeland with the centuries of Zionist yearning to recover the Jewish homeland. "Next year in

Jerusalem" sustained Jews around the world for centuries until it was realized in the creation of the Israeli state in 1948. Israeli Prime Minister Golda Meir put it this way:

> The story of modern Israel is essentially the story of the return to the ancestral homeland of exiles from persecution, insecurity, and fear in quest of freedom, human dignity, independence, and peace…. We are a people who for 2,000 years believed in the impossible. And here we are, a sovereign state.

Of course, Golda Meir also saw "a land without people for a people without land" when she looked at the territory of Palestine that became Israel.

Not surprisingly, the Palestinians found this a profoundly disrespectful vision, since they were in fact living in that land "without people" and were not willing to give up their claims. It is difficult for Americans to understand the visceral nature of this conflict. Perhaps we can do so if we look at our own response to efforts by Native Americans to reclaim their ancestral homelands. Would New Yorkers yield Manhattan to its original Indian owners? Illinois? Florida? Alaska? Oregon?

I have seen first-hand some of the feelings this sort of effort to reclaim territory produces. Along the shores of Cayuga Lake, north of Ithaca, local residents are up in arms about claims of the Cayuga Indians that they are entitled to return to or at least gain compensation for lands seized from them in the nineteenth century. Were this to be validated in the courts I would not be surprised to see violence erupt in defense of "the homeland." It certainly has happened before in America, when the interests of White America were pitted against the Native American Indian claims to the integrity of their homeland territory.

These disputes about who has a right to claim territory as their homeland affect children. Children suffer from the violence that attaches to these struggles. Children suffer from being infected with the ethnic and nationalistic hatreds fueled by conflicts over homeland. And children suffer when they do not have a clear path to positive identity. Whatever the time and place, children need a home and a homeland. Violating this right is both common in its scope and terrible in its consequences.

Case Study: Homeless Vietnamese Kids in Hong Kong's Detention Camps for "Boat People"

In 1992, I traveled to Hong Kong on behalf of a Catholic social services agency—Community and Family Service International. My mission was to conduct an evaluation of programs for Vietnamese children and youth ("boat people") who were interned in detention camps because they had arrived in Hong Kong without parents or effective guardians and without legal immigrant status. As a result, they were not allowed to become integrated into Hong Kong society or receive automatic refugee status—and thus have a right to resettlement in some other country.

The camps were spread throughout Hong Kong. This meant that reaching them required me and my colleague in the project, psychiatrist Edgardo Menvielle, to use every available form of public transportation that Hong Kong had to offer—trains, taxis, buses, and ferries. The first camp we visited required a 55-minute ferry ride. It was situated on a beautiful island—hilly, green, and surrounded by a white sand beach. It seemed rather incongruous to have a detention camp in such a luxurious site. Of all the camps in Hong Kong, this was the most open. Since it was on a carefully monitored island, people were allowed to go in and out of the compound for walks up into the hills that lie behind the fence, and to the beach (although they had to be back for roll call at the end of the day).

But the beautiful site could not hide the fact that this was essentially a prison. People were held here against their will, and all the usual issues that plague prisons were in evidence there too—fear, sexual abuse and other forms of exploitation, corruption, violence, and despair. It was like most prisons, except that it contained a broader range of the human condition, and more hope, inspiration, and decency than is typical for prisons of my acquaintance. And it sat amidst island beauty.

Inside the gates sat the compound: 10,000 people living in close conditions in a series of three-story-high "huts." Within each hut there were rows and rows of bunks, stacked three high. Each bunk was 4' × 8'. The two lower bunks had "ceilings" about 4 feet high (formed by the bunk above it), and the top bunk was open to the roof of the building. You could sit up in a bunk. There were 2 feet between the stacks of bunks in each row and about 6 feet between rows. Each family unit was assigned a bunk—a place in which to cook, store their possessions, retire to from the public areas, and sleep. The unaccompanied kids I had come to interview were typically assigned to share a bunk with one or two other people. For example, my first interview was with a 16-year-old girl who shared a third-level bunk with a 26-year-old woman who worked as a teacher's assistant in the camp school.

There was a very high birth rate in the camps. Despite close quarters, people always seem to find a way to procreate. Someone told us one reason for the high birth rate was that there had been persistent rumors that getting pregnant would improve a woman's chances of getting herself (and her family) approved for refugee status, and thus relocation. Whatever the reason, there were little kids all over the place!

I find that when it works well, the translation process almost disappears from my consciousness. I look into the eyes of the child I am interviewing and talk and listen, with the only oddity being the time delay while the translation goes into Vietnamese and the responses are changed into English. That was how well it went some days—when the translator was good. When the day's translator was bad it was slow and awkward, and I wondered how much was being lost as my words went into Vietnamese and the answers came back into English.

The second camp we visited was called She Kong. If the first camp was disarmingly like the Club Med of detention centers, She Kong was a reality check of the first order. The camp was built on an old runway—with tin-roofed Quonset huts, high barbed wire fences, and even more crowded tiers of bunks in the huts. She Kong was in the news shortly before we arrived because it was the site where a hut was burned in a dispute between two groups of Vietnamese detainees; the North–South hostility fueled by the decades of Western-sponsored war in Vietnam still has some momentum here. Twenty-two people were killed in the fire, and the trauma was widespread throughout the camp, particularly among the witnesses and those emotionally connected with the dead and injured—which included many children.

Once again, there were kids everywhere—playing within sight of the empty space in the row of huts where the burned out unit used to sit. They competed to hold my hand as we walked through the camp, and it seemed all of them have a word or two of English, mainly "hello," of course. My puppets were a bit hit with the kids as ever.

Despite its grim appearance, optimism was abroad in this camp. The staff believed the source of the optimism was that the people there had "only" been in detention for a year or so. It takes a lot of patience to be a refugee. To an outsider, the waiting seems like torment enough.

Hai Ling Chau Camp was located on a penal island. The other programs on the island have drug addicts and "regular" criminals. The detention camp itself was a former leper colony. This seemed to symbolize the status of the boat children as pariahs. It was a long, long day at Hai Ling camp because the regular translator missed the boat and I had to rely upon a paraprofessional whose English was awful. But as I think about the intellectual drudgery of that day it is balanced by my delight in being adopted for a couple of hours by a 9-year-old girl named Giap who came complete with a hula hoop. Giap allowed me to see the world of this camp through her eyes. I met her mother—and this itself was a reminder of how important it is for a child to be buffered from the dangers of the world by the loving protection of a parent. Edgardo and I both did about six interviews each day. By the end of the project I had interviewed 27 kids—and Edgardo 29—ranging in age from 9 to 18. About half the kids were truly alone, not even having a caretaker standing in place of the parents. We learned in our interviews that many were struggling with a deep sense of loss and abandonment. Two thirds indicated loss of or separation from parents prior to their departure from Vietnam, and these losses weighed heavily on the kids, for they had experienced the double whammy of losing home *and* homeland.

I recall asking one girl if she wrote to her divorced mother in Vietnam. She replied angrily, "Why should I write to her … she abandoned me." Many of the kids were on their own because one parent had died or divorced and then remarried, and the new parent rejected the "old" child and forced the remaining parent to choose between remarriage and continuing to care for the "old" child. In many cases the new husband won out over the old child (who might be as young as 5 years of age).

It came as no surprise that many of the kids we interviewed suffered from depression. They had experienced devastating losses and found themselves in chronically dangerous situations. Two thirds of them, particularly girls, told us that they spent whole days in their bunks because they were sad or depressed. Sitting with them, their sadness was often tangible. A strong sense of passivity and hopelessness was evident in many of their accounts of life in the detention camps.

Not surprisingly, we heard horrifying stories of sexual abuse from some of the girls (and indeed from some of the boys as well). At night the doors to the huts were closed; once that happened, the predatory elements took over. One girl recounted to me how several nights each week she was sexually assaulted by one of the young men who ran the hut. He would brazenly climb up to the "third-floor" bunk she shared with an older woman, demand that the older woman move to one corner of the 4'× 8' bunk, and rape the girl. She knew, as did the older woman, that reporting the young man to the camp authorities would risk violent reprisal, and was unlikely to result in him being removed from the hut.

The social realities of camp life tend to generate a pervasive apathy—just as they do in many inner city public housing projects I have visited in America. Indeed, I have often been struck by the psychological parallels of life in the camps in which internationally displaced persons live and the sites for many of America's economically displaced persons (what we often call the "underclass"). One girl told me that she often dreamed of her frequent forays into the high forests back in Vietnam to augment the family resources. She could see similar forests from the camp in which she was detained but had not left the camp once in 2 years. When she finished telling the story she sighed, laid her head on the table, and silently cried.

Two thirds of the kids I interviewed said things that told me they had given up on the future. Living in limbo, they had suspended making plans, and were unable to think beyond the present. Future orientation is critical for kids. It's what motivates them to respond positively to the various messages adults send them, which boil down to "do this now so that you can do that then." That makes sense if you see yourself in the future, but it is hollow if you don't. Kids who develop terminal thinking don't plan. And two thirds of the Vietnamese kids we interviewed in the camps evidenced just that. A depressive inertia seems to grip many of them.

Fewer than half the kids could say anything positive about life in the camps. When there was something positive, it was most likely the fact that they had a chance to go to school, something that was often better than what they had experienced in Vietnam and certainly was a diversion from their drab existence in the camp.

More than half the kids I interviewed expressed fears for their personal safety. This was particularly true of the girls—who are generally both more willing to disclose being afraid as well as being more likely to face the major threat of sexual assault. The girls spoke often of the frequent harassment they experienced, the fear they felt that older boys or men would seek to molest them in their bunks, the need they felt to make themselves as "invisible" as possible, their knowledge of rapes that had occurred, and the ever-present fear that older men would take a sexual interest in them. Some of the girls had given in to the psychological economy of the camp and admitted that they traded sexual access to one man for protection from the others. It's an ancient story for women—and is repeated in gang-infested neighborhoods across the United States as well.

Those boys who did acknowledge their fears were likely to speak of their parallel fear of bullying by older males, and the system of threats and intimidation that operated in the camps—to be sure, more in some camps than others. Many of the boys resorted to a strategy of "invisibility"—withdrawing into reading or studying, for example, as a way to avoid being noticed. This, they hoped, would reduce the likelihood of attack by predators. Like the sexual compromises of the girls, it reminded me of life in many violent inner city neighborhoods. Here too, this strategy even worked sometimes.

The camps in Hong Kong were run by the gangs, like the public housing projects I knew in Chicago in the 1980s and 1990s. Boys were recruited by "Big Brothers" who offered protection at the price of assimilation into the gang structure. For girls, there was the risk that they would enter into sexual liaisons under coercion or as a way of seeking protection.

The kids Edgardo and I interviewed were replete with traumatic experiences. Kids witnessed the violent clashes that sometimes occurred between factions. One girl spoke of her family being threatened and forced to give up all their possessions. Another child was present during the gang rape of several young women. Boys spoke of the stabbings they had witnessed. One girl entered the washroom of her hut only to find that a woman had committed suicide there by hanging herself. All the many common expressions of posttraumatic stress syndrome were evident in many of the kids as well. We found that three fourths of the kids reported terror-ridden dreams or waking at night in a state of alarm, fear, and anxiety.

One of the few comprehensive studies of these children and their fate is found in James Freeman and Nguyen Dinh Huu's 2003 book, *Voices from the Camps: Vietnamese Children Seeking Asylum*. They looked not just at the children in camps in Hong Kong, but in all the camps spread across Southeast Asia (e.g., in the Philippines, Malaysia, Thailand, and Singapore). Of the lives of children in the camps they wrote, "Taken together, these conditions show the true character of the camps: deeply abusive environments" (p. 179).

Lurking in the shadows of my memory are the images that come back more strongly when I review the stacks of photos from this trip. At High Island Camp there was a little girl who knew that her mother was in another camp in Hong Kong but because of bureaucratic red tape could not join her. Amidst the thousands of unaccompanied minors it galled me to think that this was a case so easily resolvable. I made a stink about it to the camp authorities and they were embarrassed enough to expedite the reuniting of the girl and her mother within 24 hours.

We also met with the top officials from the U.N. and the Hong Kong government responsible for the camps and the Vietnamese. Their principal interest in our findings was knowing what we had learned that could help them deal with their central problem, namely, emptying and closing the camps as soon as possible. I think the major thing we had to offer was a perspective on how the trauma experienced by the kids (and the adults) in the camps worked against the goal of getting them to take the active step of choosing to return to Vietnam.

That was the presumed fate of most of the people in the camps in 1992. Few were expected to succeed in making their cases for official political refugee status, and indeed in the years following 1992 many of the detainees were returned to Vietnam. Trauma tends to rob kids (and adults) of "future orientation," replacing it instead with a focus on the day to day. What was needed to make the decision to return was precisely the future orientation that had been taken from these kids by the traumas they had encountered (en route to the camps as well as while they detained in them).

We brainstormed with the officials about strategies to induce future orientation and thus facilitate decision making. These strategies included luring kids into future-oriented activities (everything from growing plants to writing essays to learning vocational skills). I left Hong Kong after these meetings with a grim sense of how hurt but how resilient so many of the kids were. Mostly they would survive, but the emotional scars would linger long after the governments involved finally succeeded in emptying the camps in 2001.

These children were to a great extent sacrificed on the altar of politics and the desires of adults. Their rights and needs were subordinated to the political considerations of authorities whose mission was to send as many as possible back to Vietnam so that the countries that hosted the camps could be free of them. Their rights and needs were sacrificed by parents who sometimes sent the kids on the boats in the hope of either resettling them in countries where they would be able to contribute financially to the family from afar or that they would receive payment from the international authorities for volunteering to return to Vietnam. This became a common practice in Hong Kong as the authorities became more and more desperate to empty the camps. I spoke with kids who had been sent on this perilous journey with specific instructions to accept the payments and bring the money back home so the family could start a small business.

Repatriation was the goal of the powers that ran the camps, and it justified a lot of abuse. Freeman and Huu are eloquent and forthright on this point, when they write of the abuse these children suffered:

> It was not based on economic or environmental necessity; these children were not being sacrificed so that others in the family or society might survive. The abuse they suffered was intentional, or at least permitted to continue. Officials were well aware of the violent and disintegrative environments into which these children [had] been placed … a child could end the waiting, abuse and pain; all a child need to do was offer to repatriate…. If children refused to do what they were told … then they would be punished by the removal of any remaining elements of normal childhood, such as schooling. When this did not work officials withdrew basic necessities for survival, including sufficient food and health services and in some camps deliberately relocated children in order to disrupt their lives. Abuse became the punishment for noncompliance. (p. 181)

When I next returned to Hong Kong in 2002 the camps were gone and little trace of them remained in the memories of the Hong Kong residents I spoke with about the matter. But those thousands of kids are somewhere, mostly grown up now. No doubt the most resilient have bounced back from this period when their human rights to home and homeland were violated. No doubt many suffer the emotional scars still. Freeman and Huu's follow-up analysis confirms this sad expectation. They write "While some children eventually managed to construct a decent life in Vietnam or elsewhere, including the United States, all have been scarred by their refugee experience and most are still struggling with the legacy." The lesson? No child should be alone and unaccompanied in life, whether thousands of miles away or right at home.

Chapter 9
The Right to Priority in Times of War: Would You Torture One Child to Bring World Peace?

> *Imagine that you are creating a fabric of human destiny with the object of making men happy in the end, giving them peace and rest at last, but that it was essential and inevitable to torture to death only one tiny creature—that baby beating his breast with its fist, for instance—and to found that edifice on its unavenged tears, would you consent to be the architect on those conditions?*

> —Fyodor Dostoyevsky

Since I read this passage from Dostoyevsky's, *The Brothers Karamazov*, more than four decades ago I have found it to be one of the most radical moral and political challenges in literature. For me it captures one of the most important human rights issues for children, because it seems in every war political leaders consistently answer yes to the question, "Would you consent?" They always justify and rationalize their yes vote precisely along the lines that Dostoyevsky suggested, namely, that this war is necessary because in fighting it we "are creating a fabric of human destiny with the object of making men happy in the end, giving them peace and rest at last." Just this one time, they ask, suspend your moral objections to the torture of children, in the name of the greater good, the higher principle, national honor, liberation from oppression, defense of the homeland. Just this once. And just this time. And just in this case. And so it never ends.

As the most astute students of the human condition have rightly concluded, it never can, for the fruits of torture and violence are always more violence, more children suffering with wounds to their bodies and hearts and minds. Thus, as Zen Buddhist teacher Thich Nhat Hanh so aptly puts it, "There is no way *to* peace, peace *is* the way." As Mahatma Gandhi recognized, "You must be the change you wish to see in the world." And as Jesus taught, "Do not make use of force against an evil man; but to him who gives you a blow on the right side of your face let the left be turned." (Mathew 5:39) and "Put your sword back into its place; for all who take the sword will perish by the sword." (Mathew 26:52)

And then there are the provisions of the U.N. Convention on the Rights of the Child, which speak directly to the special obligations adults have to children in times of war. Article 38 sets out the following standards for giving priority to children in times and places of war and political violence:

J. Garbarino, *Children and the Dark Side of Human Experience.*
© Springer Science+Business Media, LLC 2008

In accordance with their obligations under international humanitarian law to protect the civilian population in armed conflicts … shall take all feasible measures to ensure the protection and care of children who are affected by an armed conflict.

It also includes a mandate to exclude as soldiers youth younger than 15 years of age (a provision that has been augmented by a special agreement signed by many countries—including the United States—to set the age limit at 18).

How do we bring these principles to our concern with the human rights of children? I think ultimately we do so by putting the well-being of children ahead of any ideology or national interest and adopt a radical pacifism. Short of that, the very least we can do is be sure that we have met the U.N. Convention's mandate concerning children and war: "First do no harm."

But harm we do. Over the last century, the nature of military technology has shifted from firing individual bullets at enemy combatants to using bombs and artillery that do not differentiate between civilians and combatants. What is more, many of the wars of the last century have involved guerilla and terrorist tactics—and corresponding anti-guerilla and anti-terrorist tactics—that actually target civilians. Thus, according to UNICEF, about 90% of the casualties in modern wars are civilians, and about half of those are children.

This translates into more than 2 million dead (and 6 million permanently disabled or otherwise seriously injured) children in the 10-year period from the mid 1990s to the present. During this same period, some 20 million children have had to flee their homes and become displaced persons in their home countries or refugees, and some 300,000 were recruited—forcibly or otherwise—into the armed forces engaged in political violence in conflicts around the world.

It is said that the first law of human ecology is, "You can never do just one thing." Because human systems are so interconnected and in ways that are sometimes impossible to anticipate fully, unintended consequences, side effects, and paradoxical results are commonplace. You set out to protect children from childhood communicable diseases by inoculating them, and you end up causing an increase in autism due to the unexpected effects of the vaccine on the immune system. You set out to racially integrate schools and you end up with more segregation than you had at the outset, only now it is segregation by social class. You set out to improve the lives of poor Third World people by sending foreign aid in the form of improved farming technology, and you end up with a population explosion and land exploitation that results in widespread famine. You set out to do X and you end up with Y. This is true particularly when you set out to make war. You set out to topple Saddam Hussein and liberate Iraq, and 4 years later hundreds of thousands are dead, trillions of dollars are spent, and a civil war simmers between Sunnis and Shiites. The dead, maimed, and traumatized children are more collateral damage—just like the one tortured child posited by Dostoyevsky as the means to bring happiness and peace finally.

It is clear that war and political violence can and do hurt children, but how do they experience it psychologically? Little in the way of systematic research was conducted on the experience of children prior to World War II, and what studies were done of that conflict were informal by today's scientific standards, mostly small-scale efforts to document the emotional texture of what it meant for children to be witness to these momentous events in which ultimately 40 million civilians died. Perhaps no one has captured this as well as psychologist Emmy Werner, in her book, *Through the Eyes of Innocents: Children Witness World War II*. Werner herself grew up during World War II in Germany, and is known academically for her work on resilience. In her book she does an excellent job of representing the way children experienced the war.

Werner begins with her own memory as a 10-year-old child of September 1, 1939, the day the German Army invaded Poland:

> At dawn my mother woke me up and said, "Kind, es ist Krieg" (We are at war, my child). We sat near the radio all day, listening for news, and watched an endless parade of trains and trucks, filled with soldiers, pass by our house, heading east. When the trains stopped, we brought fruit and flowers from our garden to the men in uniform. That was Friday. On Sunday, September 3, Great Britain and France declared war on Germany. My brother was drafted the next day. (p. 7)

For American children, it was not September 1, 1939, that signaled the start of war, but December 7, 1941, with the Japanese attack on Pearl Harbor. For children in Hawaii, the attack was a physical and immediate danger. Seven-year-old Dorinda reported it this way years later:

> Suddenly we heard the sound of low flying planes, then almost immediately, loud explosions, followed by more planes passing directly over our house.... Even though we couldn't hear them, the incendiary bullets found their targets. Our kitchen was now on fire and parts of the roof were gone. Everywhere we looked there was smoke and fire. From the cane fields we could watch the skies, and if the Japanese planes came back, we could hide ourselves in the tall sugar cane stalks. I thought of the unfinished breakfast we left on the kitchen table earlier in the morning.... Maybe my dog Hula Girl had gotten so hungry that she had gotten the breakfast food. But what if she had been hit by a bomb or a bullet? It was then for the first time that I began to cry. (in Werner, p. 62)

Little Dorinda's concern for her dog's well-being is a commonality among children. Quite naturally, their very concrete minds tend to focus on the concrete effects of war—their pets, their parents, their school, their house, their world. This is not to say that children are incapable of broader concerns, beyond their immediate world.

During the Gulf War in 1991, surveys found that the most compelling images for young children were the sea birds overcome by the oil spills that were instigated by Iraqi forces as acts of sabotage and revenge in the wake of their military defeat at the hands of Allied Coalition forces. But even this testifies to the very direct and personalized nature of the way most children respond to war, most of the time. It's a point worth remembering as we consider the way modern children receive and process images and messages about war.

During World War II, children on the Mainland (where Japanese attacks were feared but never materialized in any substantial measure), responded to the news of the attack on Pearl Harbor as it came into their homes via the radio, and then were drawn into the immediate aftermath of mobilization and fear. One young teenage girl living on the West Coast put it this way:

> We were playing Christmas records when our neighbors … came running up the hill and pounded on our door. They were white as sheets and Alma was crying. Al said, "Turn on your radio, Pearl Harbor has been attacked by the Japs and we are at war." My father went to the radio and my mother slumped onto the couch with her face flushed and Alma beside her. It was obvious to me that we had been notified of a dramatic blow that had been delivered not just to Pearl Harbor, but to us individually. (in Werner, p. 63)

Jump ahead nearly 60 years to September 11, 2001 and listen to some contemporary young voices describe how they received the news that their war had begun. Dylan was 9 years old, living with his parents in Chicago on September 11, 2001. Four years later, when asked about what he remembers of that day the now 14-year-old boy offers these words, "What do I remember from 9/11? I remember the confusion and the fear I had that day. I also recollect the tears shed and the lives lost." But Dylan does not stop there. When asked what he sees in the future he says this:

> 9/11 was a horrible day in our past, but unfortunately, similar events occur every day. The terror threat towards America now is pretty strong. I mean there are people out there, filled with enough hate towards the U.S. that they'd be willing to kill themselves along with other innocent people just because they hate the U.S.A. I view the threat as high because no one will know when they'll strike or where. For example, the London terrorist attacks were completely unexpected. The terror threat towards America in the future will probably be strong or stronger.

Terrible as they were, the losses experienced by the United States in World War II were small in comparison with European and Japanese losses. Germany lost 12% of its population. The Soviet Union lost 10%. Japan lost 2%. The United States lost 0.4%. Today we must look to Iraq to see figures in any way comparable to the World War II casualties. In contrast, American civilian casualties in the war on terror have so far been small by global and historical standards, even despite the fact that the 1-day death toll on 9/11 (some 3,000 people) was greater than any other single 1-day death toll in American history. Of course, this could change once the anticipated attacks using biological, chemical, or nuclear devices actually do occur.

If massive death and destruction were not the hallmarks of the experiences of American children living through the mobilization of their democratic society in response to World War II, what were the distinctive elements? Looking backward in time we can see that it was the themes of patriotic actions in support of the war effort, efforts to balance patriotism with respect for the human qualities of the enemy, fear, and anxiety about the fate of loved ones involved directly in the conflict. Let me sample from the children's reports compiled by Emmy Werner to illustrate each of these themes.

Werner reports that:

> By the second half of 1942, Americans felt relatively secure behind their military and civil defenses…. Now the U.S. government—aided by the schools, voluntary organizations (like the Scouts, the Camp Fire Girls, and Future Framers of America), and the mass media—called

on America's children to perform a variety of patriotic tasks. Children set to work—collecting scrap, buying and selling war bonds and tending victory gardens…" (Werner, p. 67)

Even Little Orphan Annie got into the act. The daily comic strip had millions of readers among American children. In 1942, Annie saved the East Coast of the United States from a German U-boat attack. When asked by her friends why she was too busy to play with them, Annie replied:

> … I have somethin' lots more important than playin'. We're doin' war work. It's our war, just as much—or maybe more—than anybody else's. We're givin' all we can to help those who are givin' ever' thing for us! (Werner, p. 67)

Even during this "Good War" (as World War II is often called) there were struggles over finding a balance between patriotism and dehumanization of the enemy. Government and media propaganda pushed children's consciousness toward dehumanization. Japan and Germany were the enemies, but the politics of this conflict often merged into racism; particularly with regard to the "Japs." This was particularly true in the case of the 110,000 persons of Japanese descent who were summarily interned at the start of the war for reasons of "national security." Most of these were children and teenagers—two thirds of whom had been born in the United States and were thus citizens by birth. In some cases, orphans were removed from the care of orphanages, foster parents, or their teenage unwed mothers (or fathers if the father was imprisoned and the child's mother was ill or dead), and sent to specialized children's relocation centers. Manzanar was the best known of these centers and was run by an army officer who was described as a "little Hitler" by a Catholic priest who had observed his behavior in executing this odious mission.

The targets of the internment were usually forced to vacate their homes on short notice, leaving everything but what they could carry in a suitcase behind. This included pets, which must have compounded the emotional trauma for many children. The stories of this forced relocation and detention are horrifying to read half a century later for the level of emotional violence done to these innocents. Here is Werner's analysis:

> To this day, child evacuees often recall two images of their arrival at the assembly centers: a cordon of armed guards and the barbed wire and search-lights, symbols of prison. Many families arrived at the assembly centers incomplete. In some cases … fathers had been taken into custody by the FBI. (p. 82)

Of course, America was by no means uniformly bloodthirsty and racist in its response to World War II's enemies. Some mothers wrote with concern to parental advice columns about the bloodthirsty games their children played, and many teachers tried to balance out the official dehumanizing stereotypes of the enemy with pleas for tolerance, for separating the actions of governments from the humanity of the common people. One girl reported that her elementary school teacher said, "Now put yourself in their place! So many of our people are against the Germans, against the Japanese, but these people didn't make the decisions, it was their leaders" (Werner, p. 75).

But children saw the war and the enemy as a threat to their immediate emotional world and responded with aggressive images. For example, a seven year old girl wrote to her father, "If I had wings like an angel I would take some bombs and fli over to germany and japen and bom them, then you could come home sooner. I want you most of all" (Werner, p. 75).

The dominant theme for American children was fear and anxiety for loved ones fighting the war away from the American homeland. This was manifest in children's play, which is always a mirror of their emotional lives in counterpoint to the social realities they face. Children played war games relentlessly because their emotional lives were galvanized by the impact of World War II, but when the war ended they shifted back to the traditional formats of cops and robbers and cowboys and Indians. By the time I was a child in the early 1950s playing war was on a par with cops and robbers and cowboys and Indians as a safe historical topic.

What can we learn from how children and youth around the world have coped with the ongoing trauma of living with the threat and reality of political violence? I see three important themes: the limits of political ideology in giving meaning to physical suffering and injury, the allure of revenge in a situation of threat and insecurity, and the precariousness of messages of compassion amidst the struggle for homeland security unless there is a strong spiritual foundation.

All three of these principles arise from research dealing with "conventional" political violence issues—shootings, bombings, stabbings, and the like. But now we face the possibility of attacks using weapons of mass destruction—chemical, biological, and nuclear devices. There is almost no precedent for understanding how these attacks might affect children and youth psychologically and morally. There is, however, some precedent for understanding how the specter of such attacks can and does affect kids, as exemplified by the experience of insecurity children and youth faced during the Cold War and its attendant threat of nuclear attack.

Although the United States was one of the victorious countries in World War II, and emerged as the only nuclear power, any sense of security that might have derived from that status quickly evaporated as the 1940s came to an end as the 1950s began. The Soviet Union emerged as a nuclear power with the detonation of its first atomic bomb in 1949 and its first hydrogen bomb in 1953. This happened in the context of what we now know as the Cold War, in which the United States and Soviet Union contested for influence around the world and engaged in an arms race that hinged on each country's willingness to fight a nuclear war that would bring unprecedented destruction and catastrophic loss of human life.

Remember that the United States was spared the devastation experienced by the countries of Europe (and to a lesser degree Asia) during World War II, when civilians became direct targets of war in a way that they had not been for centuries. In World War I about 5% of those killed were civilians; in World War II it was 50%. Our losses were relatively small compared with the countries on whose soil the war was fought. Our cities and towns were intact. Our economy was strong and vibrant. So it was with shock that Americans in the 1950s realized that the American homeland was now vulnerable to devastating attack, that in an atomic war there would be no distinction between military and civilian, and that there were no longer going to be front lines at all, only targets for nuclear weapons.

Not since the ancient Greeks and Romans, the Crusades, the Barbarian invasions, and the Middle Ages had civilians, indeed the entire structure of day-to-day life, been the legitimate target for warriors, for whom the "sacking" of civilian population centers was considered fair game. The only American experience that could even resemble what lay ahead was the "scorched Earth" policy of the Civil War in the 1860s, exemplified by General Sherman's attack on the civilian population and infrastructure of the South.

Despite nostalgia for the relative social placidity of the 1950s (at least for the White middle-class heterosexual majority), this period was marked by the emergence of the nuclear threat, and children were aware of it. As a member of the first generation to be born into the atomic age, my own experience with duck-and-cover drills (teaching children to hide under their desks if a bright light in the sky signaled the start of an atomic attack) is testament to that. Psychiatrists and psychologists have long puzzled over the effects of this nuclear awareness on the psyche of children and youth of that period, wondering what it meant to these young minds and hearts.

Unfortunately, virtually no systematic research was conducted to answer this question. Most of the research dates from later periods—the 1970s and 1980s. But there are some fragments of information available to us that can help shed some light on how American children and adolescents are thinking and feeling about growing up in an age of terror, and how to make sense of those thoughts and feelings. Surveys of children's fears reveal that from the 1930s to the 1950s, the most common fears of children were matters of personal safety in the "old-fashioned" sense of the term, namely thunder and lightning, animals, the dark, and supernatural beings. These studies found that the fears of war rarely appeared spontaneously when children were asked about their fears. But this had shifted by the 1960s, when the most common fears became tied to political issues, most notably the Cold War and the prospect of nuclear war.

By the mid 1960s about one in five sixth graders in one study mentioned international conflicts. In 1965, a researcher asked kids how they thought the world might be different in 10 years, and 70% spontaneously mentioned nuclear war, destruction of the world, or "the bomb" in their replies.

Canadian pediatrician Susan Goldberg conducted several important studies of these issues. She found that 52% of the high school students surveyed spontaneously mentioned nuclear war as one of their three main worries. Some 58% of the teens surveyed in 1984 reported that they worried about nuclear war at least once in the previous month (compared with 64% who said they worried that frequently about job or career plans and 60% who worried about unemployment).

One very important finding in Goldberg's research that has a direct bearing on children growing up in the modern age of political violence is that the primary source of information about nuclear war was the mass media—television 74%, newspapers and magazines 60%, books 32%, and family 29%. And, although these other topics were the topic of discussions between teens and adults, nuclear war was not. Not surprisingly, kids who tended to worry a lot (daily) about jobs, career, and unemployment were also most likely to worry a great deal about nuclear war; 7% said they felt fearful and anxious every day.

There were relatively few atomic bombs in the first years after World War II, and they were of relatively small yield. Thus, devastating as atomic bombs were, they were still small enough in their destructive potential to sustain belief in protecting the civilian population with evacuation and underground bomb shelters. Thus, during the early years of the nuclear age there was serious discussion about the "survivability" of a nuclear war; after all, the only country ever to have actually been attacked with atomic bombs—Japan—had survived and had gone forward with the process of rebuilding. Indeed, I remember my sense of surprise when visiting Hiroshima in 2002 and seeing only minor traces of the atomic bomb's destruction from 1945. (During my visit even the one damaged building still standing from the attack was being refurbished to better serve as a monument.)

All this gave rise to a whole new profession, "nuclear war strategists," who concentrated on understanding the use of atomic weapons as simply big powerful military weapons, not as something unprecedented in human history, not as devices the use of which was "unthinkable." This kind of thinking reached its zenith in 1960 with the publication of Herbert Kahn's book, *On Thermonuclear War*.

But things changed quickly as both the destructive power of the weapons and their numbers and delivery systems increased exponentially in the years after 1960. In 1982 Jonathan Schell published his book, *The Fate of the Earth*, and to anyone listening, the debate about the survivability of any nuclear war—even a "limited war"—was over. It became ludicrous to see such a war as anything other than "nuclear holocaust" and "mega-death." I think awareness of this fact seeped more and more into the consciousness of American youth.

By the 1980s, about half the kids 10 and older were reporting that they believed a nuclear war in their lifetime was probable. In 2005, the figure was 60% for the entire adult population. That's not surprising, given that everyone under the age of 60 is now a veteran of the nuclear age. First this meant the Soviet threat during the Cold War. Then after a brief period of "safety" after the Soviet Union collapsed in 1991, came the era of nuclear proliferation to rogue states and the increasingly realistic possibility that terrorists would acquire nuclear weapons.

Perhaps we can see the accumulation of this shift in the finding that in 1976, 23% of high school seniors had agreed with the statement, "Nuclear or biological annihilation will probably be the future of all mankind within my lifetime," but that by 1982 the figure had grown to 35%. Some psychiatric observers see evidence of this growing awareness of the specter of nuclear annihilation in the upward trend in youth suicide and depression in the decades of the nuclear age. Indeed, a study including both American and Soviet youth in the 1980s reported that the kids who were most likely to think that a nuclear war was likely to occur were most likely to express increased pessimism about the future.

But worrisome as the threat of nuclear war is, the available evidence does not justify the belief that this fear directly produces mental health problems for most children, most of the time. After all, Japan is the only society with actual direct experience of being attacked with nuclear weapons, American weapons. Unfortunately, little is known about the mental health consequences of the attacks on Hiroshima and Nagasaki. Researchers did document many short- and long-term physical health problems resulting from these attacks, as well as social problems resulting from the stigmatization of those who survived the blasts—the Hibakusha as they are called in Japan—because of concerns about genetic effects and the low-grade long-term effects of radiation exposure such as low energy levels.

What mental health effects are evident are most likely to arise in children who are especially vulnerable. This is in keeping with the research on trauma reported in earlier chapters: The children most likely to suffer serious mental health problems from their encounters with traumatic events are the 20% of children who come to those events with emotional vulnerability or whose lives are lived with a stacked deck of accumulated risk and depleted developmental assets. Of course, psychological consequences are not the only consequences of importance. There is always the matter of philosophical and spiritual consequences.

It's important to note that realistic awareness of the threat that became the basis for action on behalf of peace was not linked to pessimism. The worst situation for kids seems to be when they are given information about the threat in such a way that both their fears and their impotence increase. Awareness coupled with constructive action may be empowering for kids—as it was for American kids in World War II, as we saw earlier.

I grew up in the nuclear age and I have traveled to many of the world's war zones. Thus, I have had first-hand exposure to societies in which children and youth have to cope with political violence. And, I have followed the research of others who have systematically explored kids' adaptations to living in each of these societies. One thing I learned from all this is that things are rarely if ever simple. The interconnection of human systems means that we can never do just one thing, and that unintended and sometimes contradictory consequences are the rule rather than the exception.

This is clear if we examine the impact of the war in Iraq on American children. One of the most clear and direct effects of the war in Iraq (and to some degree Afghanistan) has been the massive and extended global deployment of American military forces. Military mobilizations since World War II have tended to concentrate deployments among single (young) men. Due to the demographics of today's military forces (including the reliance on Reserve units), there is a disproportionate effect of this deployment on children. Today's deployments include an unusually high proportion of fathers with young children and an unprecedented number of mothers. Research documenting the effects of these deployments presents a sobering picture of the stresses these deployments impose upon families—and thus children.

It is estimated that more than 3,000 children have lost a parent to the fighting in Iraq alone. In addition, many times that number have parents who survived grievous injuries and have returned home to their families. But there is more. Rarely considered in analyzing these deployment effects is the collateral effect on the extended families of military forces—the nieces and nephews of the children of soldiers, for example. During the Gulf War in 1991, surveys revealed that almost half of America's children said they "knew" someone fighting in the war. Thus, even children who do not have a formal kinship relationship with members of the military forces can and do feel a psychological connection, a connection that opens them up to psychological effects of war trauma.

Much is said and written about globalization, about the integration of societies and communities around the world, as evidenced by shared musical tastes and trade interdependence. But the war on terror similarly has global implications for children. For example, it is estimated that 10 children died in the World Trade Centers on September 11, 2001. We mourn each child as a casualty of the terrorist's war on America. But it is estimated that America's military response cost the lives of hundreds of children in Afghanistan and tens of thousands of children in Iraq.

What is more, accounts from the region document that untold numbers of children in Iraq—and other Muslim countries in the region—have been drawn into virulent anti-American education programs. Participation in these programs could have long-lasting effects in producing an enormous number of new recruits in the terrorists' war against America, and thus bring terrorist attacks to American soil again and again and again in coming years if the political struggle is not resolved.

Of course these negative consequences are not the only effects. The American invasion of Afghanistan also meant that millions of girls started attending school who might otherwise have been denied an education because of the fundamentalist Taliban regime deposed by the American invasion. In Iraq millions of children witnessed their parents voting for the first time in free elections, and thus have had their first taste of what a democratic society might look like. A full accounting of the ripple effects of the war on terrorism is just beginning, but as has been the case in every instance of political violence in the last hundred years, children are inevitably drawn into the suffering. Protecting their rights may be an uphill battle, but it is well worth the struggle.

Case Study: Israeli Children Living with War

I first visited Israel in 1981, but my intense relationship with that country and its people really began in 1986, when I became a regular visitor and developed professional relationships with Israeli and Palestinian researchers and child advocates concerned about the effects of trauma on children. This effort resulted in several publications, and one of the most frustrating experiences of my life.

In 1991, I brought together a group of Israeli and Palestinian colleagues on the neutral ground of an American conference center for a seminar on children and political violence. My hope was that these friends and colleagues could find some common ground in a neutral setting, united by their caring for children. After 3 days the seminar ended, leaving me with tears of frustration and sadness—and perhaps a distressing sense of my own impotence in the face of such an intractable conflict.

In this, my personal experience paralleled the larger history between these two peoples. As a result of the failure of the Israeli and Palestinian leaders to find a mutually acceptable political solution to the competing claims to homeland, terrorism and war have been facts of life for Israeli children since there have been children identified as Israeli. The same goes for Palestinian children, of course, as I indicated in Chapter 5. The balance between war- and terrorism-related trauma has shifted from year to year and decade to decade as the political situation in the Middle East has itself evolved—some five wars in 50 years in counterpoint to the waxing and waning of terrorist campaigns.

In the period since September 2000 (when a new political initiative with the Palestinians failed), the predominant issue has been terrorist attacks. In a 5-year period there were almost 1,000 attacks within Israel that killed 1,042 people (nearly 20% of whom were children) and injured 7,065. In a small country like Israel (with a population of only about six and a half million, more than a million of whom are Palestinians or other non-Jewish Israelis) these numbers loom large in the consciousness and culture of the society. They are the numerical equivalent of 50,000 Americans being killed and 350,000 wounded in our population of 300 million.

Not surprisingly, most recent research focuses on the emotional impact of the terrorist attacks that have characterized this recent period in which 70% of children and youth experienced some form of terrorist attack, ranging from having stones thrown at them or people they knew to being injured or witnessing injury. Nearly 40% of Israeli children reported they knew a person who had been killed.

A survey conducted in 2002, at the time of a spike in the bombings and shootings, revealed that 27% of the kids reported mild posttraumatic stress symptoms, 10% moderate symptoms, 4% severe symptoms, and 1% very severe symptoms. These figures are lower than have been reported in other countries with crises of political violence, for example, Kuwait, Eritrea, Palestine, and Bosnia, where rates of moderate and severe symptoms ranging between 40% and 70% have been reported. Why?

The authors of the study speculate as follows:

> The lower percentage of Israeli youth suffering from posttraumatic symptoms may be attributed to the relative stability of life in Israel … the children continued to go to school fairly regularly and their parents to their jobs despite the violence. The government remained stable and, aside from occasional strikes, government services continued as before. In addition, the economic situation … was satisfactory." (p. 221)

I will testify to this personally. I am often struck by the degree to which Israelis work to create a sense of normalcy and stability for children amidst threat and danger. In a sense, it is a matter of national pride, coupled with a deep concern for the well-being of their children (setting aside the policies with regard to "enemy" children).

The U.N. Convention on the Rights of the Child pleads for just this sort of special treatment for children, this sort of social and cultural prioritizing. At least in the midst of the crisis, we can protect most children and teenagers from much of the psychological harm latent in the situation if we can minimize their exposure to risk factors beyond the violence itself and maximize their exposure to positive factors. This flows from the fact that generally it is the accumulation of risk factors in the absence of developmental assets that does the damage to children in the long run, much more so than the presence or absence of any one risk factor. But there is more to life than the absence of posttraumatic symptoms, and some researchers have looked at what it does cost Israeli children to live in a state of constant political violence.

A 1993 review called "The Effect of War on Israeli Children" includes this ominous overview by Israeli researchers Avigdor Klingman, Abraham Sagi, and Amiram Raviv:

> Israel, unfortunately, is a natural laboratory for the study of war stress. When considering war-related anxiety among Israeli children, we should keep in mind that Israeli children are brought up with a continuous awareness of war ... nearly everyone in the country knows someone who has either been wounded or died in war. (p. 75)

Recall that a survey in the United States post 9/11 indicated that 20% said they knew someone killed or injured in the attack. Imagine what these numbers would be if we had 50,000 dead and 350,000 wounded in terrorist attacks!

A review of research on Israeli children responding to the repeated war crises that have marked the first 50 years of Israel's existence reveals both resilience and adverse consequences. For example, a study of the 1973 Yom Kippur war revealed a doubling of the average level of anxiety reported by fifth- and sixth-grade children. During the 1991 Gulf War, adolescents reported high levels of stress-related responses: "refraining from taking part in pleasurable activities" (59%), "frightening images of missiles falling" (65%), "sleep disturbance" (43%), and "problems in concentration" (48%), among other symptoms of distress (p. 80). Researchers report that in general, the closer children and youth are to violent events the more these events stimulate anxiety, fear, and a variety of psychological symptoms, including depression and chronic distress. Generally, the more kids have experienced in the form of first-hand political violence the greater are their psychological symptoms, at least up to a point.

When trauma becomes chronic its effects can manifest in ways that at first glance appear paradoxical, namely less rather than more overt distress. A study of Israeli children who lived in communities close to the disputed border with Lebanon, and who thus were subject to repeated shelling from across the border, found that these children appeared to be no more anxious than kids living in similar communities far enough from the border that they never experienced shelling. The best explanation for this is that for the children living near the border, chronic shelling became a way of life, and they thus engaged in a process of adaptation (or "habituation," to use a term preferred by psychologists). Of course, this process of adaptation itself can mask deeper existential issues of meaningfulness, as well as confidence in the future and trust in adults.

We can add to this increased use of substances such as alcohol and other consciousness-altering drugs to cope with stress, according to recent reports from other Israeli researchers. This includes the finding that physical and psychological proximity to terrorist attacks in Tel Aviv was directly related to alcohol consumption by teenagers. Here there is an American parallel as well. A survey of New Yorkers in the first months after the 9/11 attacks revealed an upsurge in the use of substances linked to stress and efforts at self-soothing (cigarettes, alcohol, and marijuana). Nearly 20% of those who had not been drinking alcohol prior to 9/11 reported that they had started drinking after 9/11. Six months later there was little in the way of a return to normal for these new drinkers.

What stands against these stress-related adaptations? Religion is one counterweight. The more religious Israeli youth are, the less likely they are to use alcohol in response to the stress of living with terrorist attacks. American research reveals the same buffering effect of religion, both reducing the link between stress and alcohol use in particular and other substance abuse generally, and reducing the overall use of alcohol and other substance abuse. These effects generalize to common emotion-focused coping strategies (such as avoidance and withdrawal) in contrast to more problem-focused coping, the kind of coping that usually results in less psychological distress. Religious youth use prayer as a coping strategy rather than emotional withdrawal or deadening through the use of substances, and this generally is more positive and effective. I say generally because some studies have reported that religious youth are not better off than their more secular counterparts.

Why is this? One reason is that being "religious" is not the same for everyone. For some, being religious is mostly about a spiritual path, a way of life informed by prayer, belief, and attention to the soul. But for others, religious experience is mostly about social status and identity rather than spirituality. Psychologists studying religiosity have labeled the former an "intrinsic religious orientation" and the latter an "external religious orientation." Israeli researchers Zahava Solomon and Avital Laufer report that among Israeli youth an intrinsic religious orientation is associated with less disturbance and more emotional growth in response to the trauma of terrorism, but an external orientation is associated with less effective coping, more distress, and less emotional growth. This is a finding with extraordinary relevance to the situation of American children: It is spirituality, not the social institutions of religion, that help kids cope productively with the moral and psychological challenges of facing political violence.

Other Israeli studies tap into the role of traditional gender differences in the way children and youth respond to the threat of terrorism and war. It is often observed that girls are more expressive of their fears than are boys, who are generally taught to swallow or suppress their fears. As a result, when kids are asked to comment on their fears consciously ("What are you afraid of and how afraid are you?"), girls usually appear more fearful. But when more subtle measures, those that tap into unconscious levels of fear (what psychologists call "projective" assessments) are employed, it often appears that boys are afraid too.

Consider, for example, a study conducted by Israeli psychologist Charles Greenbaum and his colleagues of anxieties and fears related to the Gulf War and the Palestinian uprising (Intifada) in the early 1990s. Among children living in settlements in the West Bank (where Palestinians are overwhelmingly in the majority and Israeli settlements are exposed to constant hostility and threat), girls showed the highest and boys the lowest levels of conscious fears (direct answers to questions about how fearful they were). But when it came to unconscious fears and anxieties, boys were higher than girls.

Another set of findings concerns the relative impact of "normal" dangers versus the special threats posed by terrorism. Within 6 months of the end of the Gulf War (and thus the cessation of Scud missile attacks on Israel by Iraq) children were back to dealing with the "regular" threat of terrorism associated with the Intifada. At this point, children reverted to their more normal concerns, which in this case put traffic accidents at the top of the "things I worry about happening" list.

The finding that Israeli kids rate fear of traffic accidents so high is intriguing because there have been analyses of Israeli society that have linked this issue to the larger issues of threats to homeland security that are a chronic feature of Israeli life. An analysis conducted by an Israeli psychiatrist in the early 1980s, after decades of children growing up amidst the threat of terrorism and war, focused on:

> the expressions of hostility in Israeli society in reference to a broad range of daily activities (e.g., *reckless and inconsiderate driving* (emphasis added), externalization of rage towards authority figures and in general, a lack of psychological awareness and readiness to see psychological motivations in oneself and others) is an integral part of the Israeli way of life." (pp. 132–133)

If this psychoanalytic analysis is correct, one consequence of Israeli society's chronic exposure to terrorism is precisely the reckless and aggressive driving that gives rise to the traffic accidents Israeli children's fear. Following along these lines, if children felt they had a lot of conscious experience coping with the threat of terrorism and that this coping was their patriotic duty, it is not surprising that their unconscious fears should be directed at a much more socially acceptable target, namely, the violence on the highways.

When I read Moses' analysis of the displaced fear in Israeli society I thought of the young people I have known who grew up in highly violent neighborhoods in America. They too often seem emotionally "cool" ("habituated" to threat in the terms used to describe Israelis who have lived with the threat of war and terrorism). But like the Israelis in Moses' analysis, when you dig deeply you find that they also often seem hostile, psychologically dense, and impervious, even to the point of self-absorption.

The great World War II General George Patton is said to have remarked, "Compared to war all other forms of human endeavor shrink to insignificance." Hateful as it is to admit, there is more than a kernel of truth in Patton's declaration. War mobilizes a population as nothing else. It elicits cooperation and civic spirit as nothing else. The great pacifist psychologist-philosopher William James recognized this a century ago in his famous essay, *The Moral Equivalent to War*, when he wrote:

> Militarism is the great preserver of our ideals of hardihood, and human life with no use for hardihood would be contemptible. Without risks or prizes for the darer, history would be insipid indeed; and there is a type of military character which every one feels that the race should never cease to breed, for everyone is sensitive to its superiority.

But, as James so eloquently showed in his essay, the blood costs of war are so great that we desperately need a moral alternative to achieve the positive goals traditionally met by going to war. James was writing in 1906, before World War I killed eight and a half million people, World War II 55 million, and the prospect of billions dying if there is a nuclear World War III. In every past case, the war began with high hopes for speedy victory on both sides, and little appreciation of how the forces set in motion would send out ripple effects throughout each combatant society and beyond, and the number of children who would be traumatized, maimed, and killed in the process.

The bumper sticker that peace advocates often stick to their cars says, "War is not good for children and other living things." When all the rationalization is done, the truth of that statement becomes clear. Children can survive war, and can even create positive lives for themselves if given a chance to do so—by adults who put the needs of children for stability and nurturance high on their list of priorities, as the U.N. Convention on the Rights of the Child demands. But there really is no such thing as a "free lunch" when it comes to children and war. There is always a price to pay.

Chapter 10
The Right to Heal: When Traumatized Kids Need Help to Recover

Enlightenment is the ability to accept reality exactly as it is from moment to moment.

—Zen Buddhist teaching

Children have a right to heal in the wake of trauma. Protecting this right is not simply a matter of offering therapy to every child exposed to traumatic events. In fact, it may mean not offering anything but a chance to heal, and only if the child is stuck offering adult intervention in the form of therapy. It depends upon who the child is and the context in which the child is facing the prospect of recovering from trauma.

Nearly 40 years ago, when I was a counselor at a religious summer camp, there was a battered poster on the wall of the educational center that was entitled "Strong Words." It read: "Have you learned lessons only from those who admired you and were tender with you and stood aside for you? Have you not also learned great lessons from those who reject you and brace themselves against you, or who treat you with contempt, or dispute the passage with you?" I fought against the wisdom of those "Strong Words" then, but I embrace it now with the perspective of four decades more life experience.

Spiritual teachers have always recognized this truth. For example, the founder of the Jesuits, St. Ignatius of Loyola, included as a central tenet of his "spiritual exercises" the idea that our spiritual progress depends upon our ability to recognize and learn from both human life's "consolations" (the times of harmony, peace, and joy) and its "desolations" (the times of struggle, sadness, and disappointment). Buddhism teaches that suffering is inevitable in human life and the answer is not to avoid it but to embrace it as opportunity to engage in spiritual development activities that lead toward a state of enlightenment, with "non-attachment" being the necessary approach to life to achieve this state of unconditional happiness. This is one sense in which trauma offers spiritual opportunities, but it is not the only one.

One definition of enlightenment offered by a Zen Buddhist master is "to accept reality exactly as it is from moment to moment," and then to find a path that promotes caring without attachment. How can trauma contribute to this? It can do so by forcing people to see the reality of suffering in the world. What matters then is

J. Garbarino, *Children and the Dark Side of Human Experience.*
© Springer Science+Business Media, LLC 2008

what happens next. Does an individual get stuck in the horror? Or does that individual move on to enlightenment, realizing the power of love to transcend suffering? Some people get stuck, either with their fears and horrible thoughts or by drawing the conclusion that there is only negativity in the world and that in self-defense they should simply hide their heads in the sands of hedonism and sarcastic cynicism.

But learning first-hand about evil can be an inspiration to change your view of the world in a positive direction, and more actively align yourself with the power of love and good in the universe. Mentors can play a crucial role in this process. But what do children need in the short run, when trauma is most intense and prevalent? At one level, the answer is simple. After decades of professional research and intervention by social workers, psychologists, and psychiatrists, the news about dealing with and treating "simple" confrontations with horror (that is to say, one brief experience of trauma) is generally pretty good.

Put most simply, what works best in most cases is an approach that can be called the therapy of reassurance. This approach works to help children realize that things are back to normal. It is a successful intervention for most of us, most of the time, with success rates of 80% or more achieved within months of an incident. For example, 6 months after 9/11 only 10% of a sample in New York City were still experiencing the symptoms ascribed to the posttraumatic stress disorder diagnosis. Those of us who confront horror generally experience emotional disruption, but usually respond well to emotionally responsive efforts by friends and family to restore a sense of safety. When influential people in our lives don't do this we can and will feel betrayed and abandoned.

The "technology" for reassuring those who are exposed to traumatic events in the short run is well developed. We have learned important lessons from our previous experiences coping with traumatic disasters—wars (e.g., the Gulf War), natural catastrophes (e.g., earthquakes and hurricanes), school shootings (e.g., Columbine), and terrorist incidents (e.g., the Oklahoma City bombing and 9/11). These experiences offer a series of principles for responding to images of war and terrorism that flood our consciousness via the mass media. We can build upon the following conclusions drawn from past crises and challenges to provide the kind of psychological first aid that has proved effective in crisis situations around the world.

When faced with trauma most children need reassurance that they and their loved ones are safe. They need words and actions to communicate calm and safety rather than anxiety and fear. The evidence is clear that they cope best when those they look up to avoid being incapacitated by fear and anxiety. Trying to maintain regular routines is important to reassure children that normal life is not over.

There is a well-developed set of techniques for achieving a return to emotional equilibrium. It involves giving children a chance to take their time in coming to terms with the horror they have witnessed in an environment that is calm and warm. It means having sensitive and skilled mentors available to answer questions and dispel the unfounded rumors that typically begin to circulate in the wake of horror. It implies returning to comforting routines—eating regular family meals, returning to regular school schedules, maintaining normal sleep times, and the like.

These reassuring practices are sufficient for most kids, most of the time. Some professionals have formalized and extended these efforts into a package called critical incident stress management (CISM). This effort includes meeting in groups to discuss experiences, efforts to clarify information, offering a calm presence, and mobilizing family members, community organizations, and mental health professionals to help kids work through the adjustment to trauma. It was offered on a wide-scale basis to those affected by 9/11 attacks as well as to schools facing school shootings like the Columbine attack of 1999.

There are those who challenge some applications of this approach on the grounds that it can easily become a rigid formula requiring disclosure and pressuring people to re-experience trauma even when it would be in their best interest to delay confronting their overwhelming feelings and thoughts until they have stabilized their day-to-day lives. Psychologist George Bonanno is one such critic. In an article entitled, *Loss, Trauma, and Human Resilience: Have We Underestimated the Human Capacity to Thrive After Extremely Aversive Events*? Bonanno worries that the typical treatment response following traumatic events could actually undermine the adjustment of resilient persons.

Particularly when done in a heavy-handed manner, these interventions might end up insisting that an individual who appears to be coping effectively with a traumatic experience was mistaken or in denial. Breaking down the coping strategies of such resilient people would do them a disservice. Of special concern is the fact that some for-profit consulting businesses staffed with overly zealous and under-trained individuals have sprung up to offer CISM. It is in these cases that the fear that the intervention will undermine rather than promote the mental health and well-being of traumatized people seems particularly apt.

But evidence from a wide range of studies sustains two further concerns. First, even if applied in a sensitive, thoughtful, and respectful manner, the therapy of reassurance will not be enough for every child (particularly kids who have the closest connection to the horror). Second, the natural social environment of most kids does not automatically provide these elements that go beyond the therapy of reassurance—and in some cases do not even provide that much. Where either the issue arises from the special vulnerability of particular individuals or the gaps in the natural social environment itself there may well be an eventual need for more formal therapeutic interventions.

Kids already coping with loss and fear will need special reassurance. Who are they? They are kids who have family members away from home, are involved in a divorce, are hospitalized, have lost a loved one recently, or in some other way are especially worried about issues of safety, stability, and security. Everyone connected with these at-risk kids must make special efforts to offer physical, emotional, and intellectual nurturing and support. This is a major challenge, since research reveals that prior to any traumatic social event about 20% of kids in America, for example, are already troubled enough to need professional mental health services. Kids will need a chance to ask their questions and get factual information to dispel misperceptions and rumors that will arise. Friends should make themselves available to listen and then respond rather than just lecturing them on what they think is important.

When it comes to children, there are special concerns beyond these general issues. In the wake of trauma, parents and other adults will naturally tend to become preoccupied, anxious, and sad by the disaster, but they must guard against this when children are concerned. If adults are psychologically unavailable children will suffer. This is a major issue.

The message to parents is clear: Don't become glued to the television and unavailable to your children when they need you most. Parents should recognize this and remember to take time out from the news to be with their children, doing things that are reassuring. These reassuring activities include a mixture of the normal routines (to show that life goes on) and commemoration (like moments of silence and prayer and acts of service).

As they implement these general principles, what else can people do for children who have encountered horror? First, they can remember that children tend to mirror the responses of key adults in their lives. Calm and confident parents and teachers tend to produce confident children who believe the world is manageable. It is essential that parents and other adults master their fear, and communicate confidence and calm to children. Second, when communicating with children, parents and other adults should focus on positive actions that can be taken and are being taken. This includes the brave actions of adults to help victims of the tragedy, efforts of police to ensure security, and the many people who come forward to offer private help (such as donating blood).

Third, parents should try to shield young children from the most traumatic and dramatic images of violence and destruction. These images can set off significant psychological disturbance when they are intense and emotionally loaded. Remember that young children may see things in ways that are different from adults. For example, during the 1991 Gulf War, many young children were particularly disturbed by the images of the birds covered with oil from the sabotaged oil wells in Kuwait and during 9/11 some very young children thought dozens of planes had crashed into American buildings because they saw the image of the Trade Tower attack over and over, and thought each repetition was a separate event.

Fourth, parents and other adults should know that many children will feel a direct connection to the events that is not evident to adults. For example, during the Gulf War in 1991 many kids felt personally connected to the fighting, because of what to adults seemed like tangential connections. In a third grade class I studied at the time, the nephew of the children's music teacher at the school was in the U.S. Army stationed in Saudi Arabia, and the teacher had a picture of him on her desk. When asked if they knew someone fighting in the Gulf War, all of the children in the class responded in the affirmative. All these elements of psychological first aid will prove useful in helping children deal with each crisis as it comes along.

Most of the people who do not respond well to the therapy of reassurance in the wake of a traumatic event are individuals who were closest to the traumatic events and/or faced serious psychological challenges before they experienced this trauma. Why? In Burstow's terms the answer is clear: These people have already had their "cloak of invulnerability" shifted out of position (or even blown aside) by their prior confrontation with horror. Thus, for example, if there is a school shooting, the people most at risk for long-term psychological harm are those who were struggling emotionally before the incident.

Research dealing with the aftermath of 9/11 showed that among the children of New York City where the attacks took place, 6 months later nearly 30% of the children were still showing one or more signs of serious anxiety or depression, but that most of these children had been struggling prior to 9/11. Examples of these struggles include parental divorce, serious illness of a close relative, death of a pet, and especially, having been exposed to traumatic events in the past.

Being physically close to traumatic events is a predictor of the severity and durability of trauma. But being emotionally close to the events (in the sense of feeling connected psychologically to the people directly hurt) may be an even more important influence on how people respond. Indeed, the same study of New York City children cited earlier found that that "family exposure" to the attack (meaning a member of the child's family was hurt, killed, or a direct witness of the attack) was more influential in the durability of mental health problems than was the child's own direct exposure.

Among the specific procedures that have been developed over the past two decades to deal with trauma that does not succumb to the therapy of reassurance, one merits special attention, eye movement desensitization and reprocessing (EMDR). EMDR is a strategy for focusing attention while re-experiencing confrontations with horror. The key to this approach is that it provides a way to create an emotionally safe place (through the focused attention associated with directed eye movements) in which to process the arousal and cognitions that constitute the trauma in the first place. Without such a place of psychological safety the very accessing of the trauma can flood the individual with the original overwhelming arousal and cognition. With it, the process of healing can go forward.

However, there is nothing magical about the eye movements themselves. Rather, the magic of the treatment comes from the fact that it allows the brain to be calm while reviewing material that threatens to explode emotionally. Several studies have reported success with this approach for people who are stuck in their traumatic state—and who as a result may be engaging in negative behavior toward self and others, including aggression and self-medicating through drugs and alcohol.

The therapy of reassurance constitutes psychological first aid for people experiencing acute, single incidents of trauma. EMDR and other psychological therapies can help individuals who get emotionally stuck on the trauma. However, when someone experiences repeated, chronic trauma the effects are likely to be both more emotionally disruptive and to include effects beyond the immediate emotional response, issues about the very meaning of life, and spiritual and philosophical issues. This distinction between acute and chronic trauma is crucial.

One of the keys to understanding the dynamics of chronic trauma is to discriminate between the experience of trauma as "immunizing" versus "sensitizing." Immunization is the process by which a person develops resistance to an "infectious agent" as the result of being exposed to something that is derived from or similar to that infectious agent in order to allow the individual's immune system to prevent future illness when it subsequently encounters the infectious agent in question.

We are all familiar with this model. You bring your child for an injection that prevents the child from getting the mumps or polio in the future.

In the case of sensitizing, the first experience of something leads not to immunity in the future but rather to greater vulnerability. For example, consider what happens when children are hospitalized without parental presence. There does not appear to be much likelihood of serious emotional reaction to this hospitalization. The psychological effects of one hospitalization on children are usually relatively minor. It is the second hospitalization that really causes problems because rather than immunizing the child against separation anxiety the first hospitalization sensitizes the child to future separations. This is true in many aspects of human development, particularly those having to do with mental health problems.

One model involves "getting used to" the disruptive event (habituation). The other model involves becoming ever more sensitive and reactive (kindling). Kindling means that repeated exposure results in the need for less and less exposure to cause an effect. Depression seems to work like this, for example. It usually takes a major negative life event to precipitate a first depressive period, but it takes less negative stimulation to set off a second, and still less to set off a third, just as once a fire has been burning in a stove it takes less and less kindling to reignite the fire because the coals endure. In the case of kindling depression, the brain begins to adapt to the process of repeated stress in a way that makes it more and more vulnerable to arousal when challenging stimuli arrive.

So which is it in the case of trauma, immunization or sensitization, habituation or kindling? The preponderance of the evidence tells us the answer is sensitization and kindling, but with a twist. In one sense, the sensitization model is clear in the research on the effects of chronic trauma on human experience. "Prior experience of trauma" pops up repeatedly when researchers ask, "which individuals are more likely to be exhibiting distress 6 or 12 months after a potentially traumatic event?"

So what's the twist? The twist is that one of the common consequences of chronic trauma has the effect of making a person—particularly a young person— seem unaffected by future traumas. I see this all the time when I visit prisons as an expert witness to interview young men (and sometimes young women) standing trial for murder. They often seem so cool and unaffected by what they have done, what has been done to them, where they are, and what they face in the future. But are they? Of course, there are human beings who come pre-wired for coldness, for emotional disconnection. Theirs are the ranks from which psychopaths come.

A study in World War II asked, "What percent of regular soldiers become psychiatric casualties from the traumatic stress of war after six months of constant combat experience?" The answer was 98%. Who were the 2% who did not become emotionally disabled by chronic combat? They were not the most emotionally robust and psychologically healthy individuals. Rather, they were the psychopaths who experienced neither the emotional nor the moral stress of combat. Their emotional systems were locked in the "off" position and they had no moral trouble with killing. But the "normal" soldiers collapsed as the psychological and moral toll of combat exhausted their emotional resources. The good news is that most of these "normal" soldiers recovered when given sufficient rest, therapy, and the moral support of their friends, family, and fellow soldiers.

But how do "normal" soldiers cope with repeated trauma? After an initial period of anxiety—including their first combat experience—they develop a protective emotional shield to survive and keep going day after day. Until the point of breakdown they usually present as numb, cool, and detached. They do this whether they are soldiers in the army serving in Iraq or soldiers on the mean streets of violent neighborhoods. That's why the young men I see in court are so cool. Mostly they are not psychopaths (although some are). Mostly they are chronic trauma cases that have not yet reached the point of collapse.

So where does their trauma go, if not into the kind of overt disturbance and upset that is so common for first-time trauma victims in the immediate aftermath of their horrible experience? It goes inside in the form of nightmares. It goes into the abuse of substances as a form of self-medicating. It gets displaced into rage that diverts energy from sadness. It goes into the way their brain functions when aroused. It gets attached to fears that deflect attention from the primary fear. If we look for it we can find it in many places that at first glance seem like psychological red herrings.

Looking at the issue of trauma as a threat to the human rights of kids we come up with three principal conclusions. First, trauma follows a sensitization rather than an immunization model. In general, an initial trauma creates greater vulnerability to subsequent traumas. Second, psychological realities put some people at heightened risk in comparison with others, most notably from their susceptibility to overwhelming arousal and their relative defenselessness in the face of overwhelming negative cognitions. Third, people differ in the degree to which they are vulnerable to the negative effects of trauma. Some are hardier than others.

Just knowing these three things about the way people experience trauma is a good start to knowing where to look when we search for ways to support the human rights of kids living in the shadows of the dark side of human experience. The right to feel safe is primal and it is a right abridged all too often.

Safety flows from a feeling of security. Of course we as adults know that there is danger in the world. We know that there is cancer, that there are serial killers loose among us, that there are bands of terrorists around the world who hate America; in short, that horrible things happen every day. But we also know that children need childhood. They need to be sheltered from the dark side of life until they have grown strong enough to recognize it and not be traumatized by it. This is the task for adults, and it is sometimes more than adults can handle.

Case Study: Children in Kuwait and Iraq: Sacrificing Children to the Needs of Adults

The issues of healing trauma come to a head when kids are engulfed in situations of violence. I saw this when I traveled on behalf of UNICEF to Kuwait and Iraq in the wake of the Gulf War in 1991. One of the most important lessons to be drawn from those experiences concerns the difficulties adults often have seeing and acknowledging the impact of trauma on children. This takes several forms. One is the strong motive we all have as parents who care for children to believe things are "back to normal" for traumatized children as soon as possible. Of course, children sometimes collaborate in this deception.

Who wants to be defined by victimization? Most children don't, and few adults want that either. The pressure from within the child and from outside to "get over it" is strong. I saw that in the families in Kuwait just days after the war's end—and I have elsewhere. The horror a parent feels when confronted with a traumatized child, the helplessness, the powerlessness can be overwhelming. How emotionally useful it is for parents to believe that their children are not permanently harmed by what they have experienced!

This emotional difficulty is compounded by the fact that many children mask their symptoms of trauma. Over time (particularly after 6 months) children may deliberately or unconsciously hide symptoms of trauma to reassure concerned adults and avoid being labeled as abnormal. I recall talking with my psychiatrist friend Bruce Perry about his observations of the children who survived the Branch Davidian catastrophe in Waco, Texas in 1993. He said that when he first met with the children they seemed normal on the surface. Indeed, prior to his visit, the local mental health professional had been in to see them and pronounced them OK. Being both more expert in understanding the dynamics of trauma, and a more incisive observer of children, Perry knew this apparent OK-ness was improbable. After all, these children had lived with the demonic David Koresh, and had endured the FBI–ATF siege on the compound. So Bruce did more than look. He measured the resting heart rate of the children (which under normal circumstances would be expected to be about 78 beats per minute) and found the average rate was 148. All this made perfect sense to me in Kuwait and Iraq. But there was more.

What I saw a great deal of in Kuwait and Iraq was adults appropriating the experience of children for their own purposes. In both cases this was often political. It served the political interests of Kuwait to acknowledge the trauma experienced by children in the short run, but to deny it in the long run. This added to the moral weight of victimization that provided the principal rationale for Kuwaiti efforts to explain the Gulf War to themselves and others. The sense of simple victimization and outraged innocence in Kuwait was nearly omnipresent. "How could they do this to us?" people asked me. And even more telling was the Kuwaiti disbelief that anyone else in the Arab world could have supported the Iraqi invasion or felt a smug sense of Kuwait having deserved the invasion as punishment for its past arrogance.

The need to rationalize their experience eventually took the form of children in Kuwait being shown videos of Iraqi atrocities to "prove" how bad the Iraqis were, and simplistic explanations of the invasion and occupation based upon the theme "the Iraqis are bad." These messages were simple, but devastating for the many Kuwaiti children of mixed Kuwaiti–Iraqi marriages. What is more, therapeutic resources for Kuwaiti children were often not made available (e.g., not opening the schools or providing some similar group experiences for kids soon after the liberation, as was at the heart of my recommendations for UNICEF).

The political appropriation of children's suffering was worse still in Iraq. Once again, in the short run this took the form of belligerently proclaiming the trauma of children—often parading children in front of cameras—but only as political instruments to castigate the United Nations and United States for the economic sanctions imposed to put pressure on Saddam Hussein's regime. The professionals I spoke with—often pleaded with—in Iraq to mount a therapeutic campaign, even to accept U.N. resources to mount such a campaign, uniformly stonewalled.

Why? Because they said there was nothing to be done for children so long as the U.N. sanctions were in place. And that their faith in Uncle Saddam was therapeutically enough in the absence of international justice. Although for different motives, here again was political appropriation of the suffering of children for adult purposes.

In the case of Kuwait, I returned twice to help deal with the psychological damage left behind by the invasion, occupation and war. On both visits—6 months and 1 year after liberation—the dominant theme was the unresolved trauma issues facing children. In the case of Iraq, I have not returned. (I planned to do so in 2003, until insurgents blew up the U.N. headquarters in Baghdad and those plans were destroyed with the building.) But all indications from others who did return are that the political intransigence of Saddam Hussein's regime and its political appropriation of the suffering of children continued unabated over the years and were ended only with the fall of the regime in April 2003. Saddam Hussein's regime is gone, and the chaotic processes of change is underway with widespread insecurity the rule rather than the exception. The precise consequences for Iraq's children are unknown, but there are widespread reports of chronic and massive trauma among Iraqi children and the political violence has continued year after year. Whether it is Kuwait or Iraq, it is business as usual for a society that will never be the same as it was.

What is the lesson in all this? Children have a right to their suffering and a legitimate claim to the time and resources it takes to recover from trauma without adults laying claim to it for their own purposes. They have a right to heal. What are the barriers to the responsiveness that children need in the face of trauma?

They may flow from the parent's personality—notably self-absorption and self-centeredness (narcissism). But they may also arise through parental emotional unavailability precipitated by crisis in the parent's life as an adult—for example, separation and divorce, in "normal" times and the exigencies of political violence in "abnormal" times such as the present.

For example, my own research with Palestinian children showed us that in conditions of threat and terror children do best when they face these threats in the context of warm and supportive families. These are families in which parents listen to children and permit them to enter into a positive dialogue about the meaning of political events, rather than silencing them or punishing them for their fears and anxieties. I saw evidence of this as well in Kuwait after the Gulf War of 1991. Parents who were emotionally open to their children did a better job of helping those children manage the trauma of the Iraqi occupation.

Studies from around the world—including North America—document that parents who are able to see and hear the feelings of their children and respond respectfully and warmly to these feelings are most likely to produce emotionally healthy children. Whatever its origins, empathic parenting is particularly important when children are facing difficult life circumstances such as the trauma of living with the reality of terrorist attack.

Director Steven Spielberg acknowledged in an interview that he approached making the 2005 film "War of the Worlds" differently because of 9/11 than he would have before. But there was more to the interview than this point. Spielberg recalls the 1951 science fiction film "Invaders from Mars" as the most disturbing of the many such films he viewed as a child. Why? Because in the film aliens tamper with a young boy's parents—implanting devices in their necks that allow the aliens to control and manipulate them and in so doing turn them away from their child.

As Spielberg sees it, this is the primal fear of childhood, that your parents are not your parents, that they will turn away from you because they are under the control of alien forces. This is why "Invasion from Mars" worked. It is why Spielberg saw it five times. I saw it twice. It left indelible memories for both of us, memories that as an artist Spielberg can employ as creative inspiration while I can only use them to stimulate my compassion for today's children.

The 1950s could be a scary time for sensitive children, what with the repeated warnings of the impending atomic doom that we received from our parents, our teachers, the burgeoning science fiction movie genre, and some of our political leaders. What we needed then (but mostly did not receive) and what children need now (and may well be more likely to get in our much more psychologically sophisticated era) was and is intelligent empathy on the part of parent, and teachers, and every other adult in the lives of children, for that matter.

Children look to parents and other key adults in their lives for cues and clues about what to make of powerful events that come to them via the mass media and even directly from their observation of events in their immediate environment. This is one of the most important influences parents and teachers have on the children they care for and educate. The child's understanding of the world is very concrete. For a child, the most powerful question is "How is my world?" They have a right to all the time and support it takes to heal their view of the world, on their own behalf, without being appropriated or managed by adults with their own agendas.

Epilogue

The Right to Joy and Happiness
and the Life of the Spirit

Let me begin with a parable—a teaching story—about the role of spirituality in the process of searching for a higher moral calling in the face of fear and uncertainty. I call it the parable of the lamp post. A friend of ours, let's call him Joe, is on his way home one dark night when he encounters his friend George, on his hands and knees groping around on the ground under a lamp post. "What's the matter?" asks Joe. George responds, "I've lost my car keys and I live 35 miles away and I can't go home until I find them." "Let me help you," Joe replies, and like a good American neighbor he too begins groping around on the ground under the lamp post.

They don't find the keys, so eventually, Joe suggests they take a new approach, a psychological approach. He says, "Now George, let's try a behaviorist psychology approach. I'll use these M&Ms to reinforce your 'key-seeking behavior.'" He does so but they don't find the keys. "Hmmm," says, Joe. "That didn't work. Let's try a psychodynamic/psychoanalyatic approach." So he begins asking George about early losses in his life and eventually George recovers the memory of having lost his teddy bear when he was 5 years old, and realizes that the loss of the keys is tapping into the feelings associated with the loss of his teddy bear. So they process George's loss issues, and eventually George gains insight. But he can't go home because he still doesn't have the keys.

"Well," says Joe, "let's try a cognitive developmental therapy approach." And he begins to explore flaws in George's concept of "keyness" and its relation to self. This too fails to produce the keys, although George emerges with a much clearer concept of the keys he does not have in hand. This having failed, Joe suggests a support group, he opens his cell phone and calls other people who have lost their car keys and has George talk with them. Soon George is feeling OK about losing his keys. But he still can't go home. Finally, Joe says, "Conventional psychology is not enough. Let's take a radical approach: Where exactly were you when you lost the keys?"

George answers, "About 100 yards down the road." Joe is stunned and asks, "So why are we looking here?" With fear George looks up the road and says, "Because the light is much better here and I'm afraid of the dark." Hearing this, Joe smiles and says, "Well then, take my hand, let us pray and then we will walk together into the darkness."

I have thought of that parable often in my professional life, where over the last 30 years I have had many opportunities to walk into the darkness—war zones, refugee camps, abusive families, violent neighborhoods, prisons, and death row. And I think of it often as I watch the news of more terrorist attacks and violent reactions to those attacks, more abused and neglected children, more impoverished and exploited families, and more suffering from natural and human-created disasters in all its myriad forms. I think of this parable so often because I know that to deal with the assaults on the human rights of children that occur on the dark side of human experience we need to bring to bear more than only the conventional tools of psychology. I have found I must adopt a spiritual orientation if I am going to learn the most important lessons that these experiences can teach. What are those lessons about what matters most in the lives of children and the adults who care for them?

The first lesson is that the experience of injustice offers spiritual opportunities just as it offers moral challenges. What determines whether we seize and profit spiritually from these experiences or allow them to feed the dark side of human selves, our needs to be powerful, in control, and angry? If we knew that and could bottle it the world would be a very different place. But it is not enough to say that much and give up with a feeling of resignation, sadness, or despair. I think there are some answers to that question. They come from all three forms of human knowing: science/humanities, human studies, and soul searching.

From science and humanities we learn that the more a child is surrounded and supported by positive people who demonstrate caring and love for that child the more likely it is a child will walk into the light rather than embrace the darkness. The world of ideas can offer resources of children facing trauma and danger and these children have a right to access the noblest and most inspiring elements of culture that can be made available. For these children, the arts are not a luxury but rather a basic necessity, for example. For these children beauty and noble role models are often a matter of basic moral and psychological survival. Of course, the more conventional resources for functional resilience are needed as well—educational opportunities, supportive social relationships, at least average intellectual ability, androgyny, and the like.

From human studies we learn that children facing danger and trauma need the opportunity and encouragement to tell their story and to have someone listen. Even though the listener cannot have total empathy (intersubjective transmissibility, to use that awkward technical term), the listener can provide a fertile environment in which the individual child can best go about the business of making peace with their unique experience. What differentiates kids with lousy early lives who go on to live good later lives from kids with lousy early lives who live lousy later lives is often precisely this ability to create a positive narrative from their encounter with darkness, danger, and trauma.

Finally, from soul searching we learn that human consciousness has the capacity to experience the sublime of the divine. Buddhism and Christianity offer how-to manuals for this purpose. Meditation and meditative prayer provide a vehicle for transcending suffering. Indeed, in many ways that is what they were explicitly created to do. Evidence mounts that this practice can actually change the human brain, enhancing the areas of the brain that are associated with concentration and happiness. When Buddhism says "Enlightenment is accepting reality exactly as it is in every moment" it is teaching not a sour resignation, but a liberating happiness. Just look at the face of the Dalai Lama or Thich Nhat Hanh and you can see how their practice transforms the heavy suffering in their lives (the loss of his homeland in the case of the Dalai Lama and the loss of several generations of countrymen to warfare for the Vietnamese Thich Nhat Hanh). Similarly, when Christianity teaches that Jesus died for our sins and thus that everyone can find the path to heaven through faith and goodness it provides an equally liberating path from the suffering of the dark side of human experience.

Protecting the human rights of children requires that the advocate be prepared to employ all three ways of knowing. It requires the tough-minded practice of scientific theory and research as well as the dispassionate exploration of cultural resources. It requires a willingness to be there with those who experience the dark side of human experience, to listen to them and help them craft a positive personal narrative. And, it requires that all this worldly work be done from a position of spiritual strength, from daily practice—meditation and prayer.

The satiric humorist of the 1920s, H.L. Mencken once wrote: "There is always an easy solution to every human problem – neat, plausible, and wrong. Americans yearn for simplicity and distrust complexity. But in many ways the world is not obliging; complexity and paradox are common, and things are often not what they seem. We need all three ways of knowing to do the right thing.

What we do matters in our own lives, in the larger world, and for the future. It matters in our public policies, social programs, and sense of ourselves as moral beings. It matters to our ability to live a soulful existence, one that meets our spiritual needs. And this is all the more reason for us to have the deepest, most sophisticated analysis of the issues that confront and surround us as we seek to nurture the human rights of kids.

One last note. I have approached these issues both as a scholar and as a person of faith. Belonging as I do to a Jesuit University community (Loyola University Chicago) I see no contradictions between these roles. Indeed, it is a foundational principle of my Jesuit colleagues and mentors that people of faith need not fear science and reason, because we believe we find "God in all things." The world is as it is and God infuses it in every aspect.

Acknowledgements I want to thank the many people near and far who have helped and supported me in this work. First among them is my wife Claire Bedard, Whose insight and inspiration flow through me in these pages. Second, I thank my graduate research assistant at Loyola University Chicago—Eddie Bruyere—who has provided great technical and moral support in preparing this manuscript. I also thank the students over the years who have responded to the ideas contained in this book—most notably the graduate and undergraduate students in my Fall 2007 course at Loyola ("A Developmental Perspective on the Human Rights of Children"), who read the manuscript and much of the supporting documentation and who showed courage in looking directly at the lives of children facing the dark side of human experience.

References

1 *Sword and the Chrysanthemum.*: Benedict, R. (1989). *The Chrysanthemum and the sword: Patterns of Japanese culture.* Boston: Mariner Books.

1 **this when he wrote:** Xenien aus dem Nachlass #45

2 **peoples of the South Pacific.:** Mead, M. (1935). *Sex and temperament in three savage tribes.* New York: William Morrow.

2 **Nineteenth century Frenchman de Toqueville's:** de Tocqueville, A. (1904). *Democracy in America.* New York: D. Appleton and Company.

3 **rejection a "psychological malignancy.":** Rohner, R.P. (1975). *They love me, they love me not: A worldwide study of the effects of parental acceptance and rejection.* New Haven, CT: Human Relations Area Files Press.

3 **practical as a good theory.:** Lewin, K. (1952). *Field theory in social science: Selected theoretical papers by Kurt Lewin.* London: Tavistock.

4 **one vessel to another.:** Shaffer, David B. (2006). *Developmental psychology*, 7th ed. Belmont, CA: Wadsworth.

4 **immature in young adolescents.:** Yurgelun, T.D. (2002). Frontline interview available at http://www.pbs.org/wgbh/pages/frontline/shows/teenbrain/interviews/todd.html

4 **18% of teenagers and adults.:** Davidson J., & Smith R. (1990): Traumatic experiences in psychiatric outpatients. *J Trauma Stress* 3:459–475.

4 **child or group of children.:** Garbarino, J., & Bedard, C. (2001). *Parents under siege: Why you are the solution, not the problem, in your child's life.* New York: Touchstone.

5 **the eyes of that child.:** Bronfenbrenner, U. (1972). *Two worlds of childhood: U.S. and U.S.S.R.* New York: Simon & Schuster.

5 **Psychoanalyst Bruno Bettelheim:** Bettelheim, B., & Rosenfeld, A. (1993). *The art of the obvious: Developing insight for psychotherapy and everyday life.* New York: Knopf.

5 **"ecological perspective" on human development.:** Bronfenbrenner, U. (1970). *The ecology of human development: Experiments by nature and design.* Cambridge, MA: Harvard University Press.

6 **almost always "it depends.":** Garbarino, J. (1992). *Children & families in the social environment.* Piscataway, NJ: Transaction Publishers.

6 **girls but not in boys):** Maccoby, E.E., Dowley, E.M., Hagen, J.W., & Degerman, R. (1965). Activity level and intellectual functioning in normal preschool children. *Child Development* 36(3):761–770.

6 **supportive and long term intervention):** Thomas, A., & Chess, S. (1977). *Temperament and development.* New York: Brunner/Mazel Publisher.

6 **time better than children):** Shaffer, David B. (2002). *Developmental psychology*, 7th ed. Belmont, CA: Wadsworth.

6 **the figure is 15%):** Loeber, R., & Farrington, D. (1999). *Serious and violent juvenile offenders: Risk factors and successful interventions.* Thousand Oaks, CA: Sage.

6 **than a source of pride:** Garbarino, J., & Ebata, A. (1983). The significance of ethnic and cultural differences in child maltreatment. *Journal of Marriage and the Family* 45(4):773–783.

6 **Psychologist Mavis Hetherington's book:** Hetheringtons, E.M., & Kelly, J. (2003). *For better and for worse: Children of divorce.* New York: W.W. Norton.

7 **babies the figure was 10%:** Thomas, A., & Chess, S. (1977). *Temperament and development.* New York: Brunner/Mazel.

7 **Research conducted by the Search:** Lerner, R.M., & Benson, P.L. (2002). *Developmental assets and asset-building communities: Implications for research, policy, and practice.* New York: Kluwer Academic/Plenum.

7 **of overwhelming risk accumulation.:** Tolan, P. (1996). How resilient is the concept of resilience? *The Community Psychologist* 29:12–15.

8 **with internalized symptoms of distress.:** Rutter, M. (1989). Pathways from childhood to adult life. *Journal of Child Psychology and Psychiatry* 30:23–51.

8 **for better and for worse.:** Perry, B.D., Pollard, B.A., Blakley, T.L., Baker, W.L., & Vigilante, D. (1995). Childhood trauma, the neurobiology of adaptation, and "use-dependent" development of the brain: How "states" become "traits." *Infant Mental Health Journal* 16(4):271–291.

8 **well being and survival,:** Garbarino, J. (1995). *Raising children in a socially toxic environment.* San Francisco: Jossey-Bass.

8 **Law Professor Michael Perry,:** Perry, M. (2006). The morality of human rights. *Commonweal* 133(13):16–18.

Chapter 1

9 **never completely account for outcome:** United States Census Bureau (2002). International population reports WP/02: Global population profile. Retrieved February 18, 2007 from http://www.census.gov/ipc/prod/wp02/wp-02.pdf

10 **the area of the church:** Horwitz, S., & Ruane, M. (2004). *Sniper: Inside the hunt for the killers who terrorized the nation.* New York: Ballantine Books.

11 **scholars have called human studies:** Cohler, B. (1991). The life story and the study of resilience and response to adversity. *Journal of Narrative and Life History* 1(2–3):169–200.

12 **"inter-subjective transmissibility.":** Husserl, E. (1970). *The crisis of European sciences and transcendental phenomenology.* David Carr, trans. Evanston, IL: Northwestern University Press.

12 **"in the present moment.":** Hanh, T.N. (1999). *The miracle of mindfulness.* Boston: Beacon Press.

13 **"finding God in everything and everyone,":** Basic tenets of Jesuits available at www.jesuit.org

13 **Similarly, whether you are the:** Saint Ignatius of Loyola, & Tylenda, J. (2001). *A pilgrim's journey: The autobiography of St. Ignatius of Loyola.* Ft. Collins, CO: Ignatius Press.

13 **Similarly, whether you are the:** Teresa, M. (1997). *Mother Teresa: In my own words.* New York: Gramercy.

13 **Similarly, whether you are the:** Hanh, T.N. (1999). *The heart of the Buddha's teaching.* New York: Broadway.

13 **Similarly, whether you are the:** Lama, D. (2006). *The universe in a single atom: The convergence of science and spirituality.* New York: Broadway.

13 **"soul traveling":** Holland, R., Hultkrantz, A., & Hultkrantz, A. (1997). *Soul and Native Americans.* Putnam, CT: Spring Publications.

13 **see the path in prayer.:** Gaskins, P.F. (2004). *I believe in … Christian, Jewish, and Muslim young people speak about their faith.* Peru, IL: Cricket Books.

13 **Hindus speak of insight meditation.:** Kamalashila (1997). *Meditation: The Buddhist way of tranquility and insight.* Birmingham, UK: Windhorse Publications.

13 **Hindus speak of insight meditation.:** Malhotra, A.K. (1993). *On Hindu philosophies of experience: Cults, mysticism and meditations.* SUNY Binghampton University: Global Publications.

14 **leader in teaching about compassion.:** Lama, D. (2001). *An open heart: Practicing compassion in everyday life.* New York: Little, Brown and Company.

14 **"Love thy neighbor as thyself.":** Stott, J.R. (1993). *The message of the sermon on the Mount.* Downers Grove, IL: Inter-Varsity Press.

15 **"No Man is an island/no man stands alone.":** Donne, J. (1624). *No Man is an island/no man stands alone,* in Meditation VVII.

Chapter 2

17 **"for evil in human nature.":** Sgroi, S. (1988). *Evaluation and treatment of sexually abused children and adult survivors. Vulnerable populations.* New York: Free Press.

17 **Perhaps the most powerful simple:** Garbarino, J. (1996). The spiritual challenge of trauma. *American Journal of Orthopsychiatry* 66:162–163.

17 **As psychiatrist Bruce Perry:** Perry, B.D., Pollard, B.A., Blakley, T.L., Baker, W.L., & Vigilante, D. (1995). Childhood trauma, the neurobiology of adaptation, and "use-dependent" development of the brain: How "states" become "traits." *Infant Mental Health Journal* 16(4):271–291.

18 **research by psychologist George Bonnanno:** Bonanno, G.A. (2004). Loss, trauma, and human resilience: Have we underestimated the human capacity to thrive after extremely adverse events? *American Psychologist* 59:20–28.

19 **was not until decades later:** Op Den Velde, W., Pelser, H.E., & Frey-wouters, E. (1994). The price of heroism: Veterans of the Dutch Resistance to the Nazi occupation and the Holocaust in World War II. *Holocaust and Genocide Studies* 8(3):335–348.

19 **infrequently rather than being constant.:** Myers, D. (2004). *Psychology.* New York: Worth Publishers.

19 **"an event from which you never fully recover.":** Garbarino, J., Dubrow, N., Kostelny, K., & Pardo, C. (1992). *Children in danger: Coping with the consequences of community violence.* San Francisco: Jossey-Bass.

20 **conducted by psychiatrist Kenneth Fletcher.:** Fletcher, K. (2003). Childhood post traumatic stress disorder. In E.J. Mash and R.A. Burkley (eds.), *Child psychopathology,* 2nd ed. New York: Guilford.

20 **Psychologists Davidson and Smith found:** Davidson, J., & Smith, R. (1990). Traumatic experiences in psychiatric outpatients. *J Trauma Stress* 3:459–475.

20 **ages of 6 and 11.:** Erickson, K. (1978). *Everything in its path: Destruction of community in the Buffalo Creek flood.* New York: Simon & Schuster.

21 **agree with psychiatrist Lenore Terr:** Terr, L. (1995). *Unchained memories: True stories of traumatic memories, lost and found.* New York: Basic Books.

21 **inhabiting adolescent or adult bodies.:** Garbarino, J. (1999). *Lost boys: Why our sons turn violent and how we can save them.* New York: Anchor.

22 **in a gang-related shooting.:** Terry, D. *Even a grade school is no refuge from gunfire.* The New York Times, 1992.

22 **Stanley Milgram was a Yale:** Myers, D. (2004). *Psychology.* New York: Worth Publishers.

22 **"for a good purpose.":** Milgram, S. (2005). *Obedience to authority.* London: Pinter & Martin Ltd.

23 **of what they were experiencing.:** Lindy, J.D. (1987). *Vietnam: A casebook.* Levittown, PA: Brunner/Mazel.

23 **psychotherapist Bonnie Burstow argues that:** Burstow, B. (2005). A critique of posttraumatic stress disorder and the DSM. *Journal of Humanistic Psychology* 45(4):429–445.

24 **Traumatic events can be the:** Fredrickson, B.L., Tugade, M.M., Waugh, C.E., & Larkin, G.R. (2003). What good are positive emotions in crises? A prospective study of resilience and emotions following the terrorist attacks on the United States on September 11th, 2001. *Journal of Personality and Social Psychology* 84(2):365–376.

26 **elicit traumatic responses in children:** Nader, K.O., Pynoos, R.S., Fairbanks, L.A., al-Ajeel, M., & al-Asfour, A. (1993). A preliminary study of PTSD and grief among the children of Kuwait following the Gulf crisis. *British Journal of Clinical Psychology* 32:407–416.

26 **Space Shuttle Disaster in 1986:** Terr, L.C. (1991). Childhood traumas: An outline and overview. *American Journal of Psychiatry* 148(1):10–20.

26 **children psychologist Joanne Cantor's:** Harrison, K.S., & Cantor, J. (1999). Tales from the screen: Enduring fright reactions to scary media. *Media Psychology* 1(2):97–116.

26 **away from New York City.:** Whalen, C.K., Henker, B., King, P.S., Jammer, L.D., & Levine, L. (2004). Adolescents react to the events of September 11, 2001: Focused versus ambient impact. *Journal of Abnormal Child Psychology* 32:1–11.

Chapter 3

29 **falsehood is worse than death.:** Boyce, M. (2001). *Zoroastrians: Their religious beliefs and practices.* London: Routledge.

29 **family, work, and the community.:** Garbarino, J. (1995). *Raising children in a socially toxic environment.* San Francisco: Jossey-Bass.

30 **10–15% of the variation.:** The American Psychological Association's 2001 report: Anderson, C., et al., "Influences of media violence on youth."

30 **"....general social or vocational capabilities":** American Psychiatric Association (2000). *Position statement: COPP Position Statement on Therapies Focused on Attempts to Change Sexual Orientation (Reparative or Conversion Therapies).* Retrieved on February 04, 2007 from http://www.psych.org/psych_pract/copptherapyaddendum83100.cfm

30 **after a fight at school:** Garofalo, R., Wolf, C., Kessel, J., Palfrey, J., & Durant, R.H. (1998). The association between health risk behaviors and sexual orientation among a school based sample of adolescents. *Pediatrics* 101(5):895–902.

31 **is today among college students.:** Comstock, D. (1991). *Violence against lesbians & gay men.* New York: Columbia University Press.

31 **are homosexual in their orientation:** The Kinsey Institute (1999). *Prevalence of homosexuality.* Available at www. Kinseyinstitute.org

31 **come out to their parents:** Garbarino, J., & Bebard, C. (2001). *Parents under siege: Why you are the solution, not the problem, in your child's life.* New York: Touchstone.

31 **leaders, and other public figures.:** MSNBC.com (Jan 22, 2007). ABC rebukes *'Grey's Anatomy' star for slur: 'I can neither defend nor explain my behavior,'* says Isaiah Washington. Retrieved on February 12, 2007 from http://www.msnbc.msn.com/id/16696521/

31 **leaders, and other public figures.:** Media Matters for America. *Robertson: Gays and lesbians are "'self-absorbed narcissists'" responsible for no-fault divorce and abortion* (August 17, 2005). Retrieved on February 05, 2007 from http://mediamatters.org/items/200508170006

31 **change his or her sexual orientation.:** American Psychiatric Association (2000). *APA Position Statement on Psychiatric Treatment and Sexual Orientation December 11, 1998.* Retrieved on February 04, 2007 from http://www.psych.org/psych_pract/copptherapyaddendum83100.cfm

32 **... the mall again," he replied.:** Garbarino, J. (1999). *Lost boys: Why our sons turn violent and how we can save them.* New York: Anchor.

32 **neighborhoods the figure is 60%!:** Loeber, R., & Farrington, D. (1999). *Serious and violent juvenile offenders: Risk factors and successful interventions.* Thousand Oaks, CA: Sage.

32 **adolescent drug abuse became epidemic.:** Kelly, J.A., & Amirkhanian, Y.A. (2003). The newest epidemic: a review of HIV/AIDS in central and eastern Europe. *International Journal of STD & AIDS* 14(6):361–371.

32 **the Philippines is child prostitution.:** Mulhall, B.P. (1996). Sex and travel: studies of sexual behaviour, disease and health promotion in international travellers-a global review. *International Journal of STD & AIDS* 7(7):455–465.

32 **violence became epidemic in Colombia.:** Wadlow, R. (2002). *Violence in Columbia, 1990–2000: Waging war and negotiating peace.* St. Paul, MN: Professors World Peace Academy.

33 **responsibility, fairness, caring, and citizenship.:** Lickona, T. (2004). *Character matters: How to help our children develop good judgment, integrity, and other essential virtues.* New York: Touchstone.

34 **many residents of the city.:** Briscoe, D. (2007). *Katrina: A systematic failure.* Retrieved on September 07, 2007 from http://www.msnbc.msn.com/id/20546339/site/newsweek/

34 **point it has reached today.:** Garbarino, J., Kostelny, K., & Dubrow, N. (1991). *No place to be a child: Growing up in a war zone.* New York: Lexington Books.

34 **the Rights of the Child:** Bedard, C. (2007). *Children's rights are human rights.* Chicago: Loyola University Press, Center for the Human Rights of Children.

34 **"historical exceptionalism.":** Kaplan, S.J., Pelcovitz, D., & Fornari, V. (2005). *The treatment of children impacted by the World Trade Center attack.* New York: Hawthorn Press.

35 **Kuwait and threatened Saudi Arabia:** Bennis, P. (2002). *Before and after: US foreign policy and the September 11th crisis.* New York: Olive Branch Press.

35 **matter of access to petroleum:** Simons, G. (2004). *Iraq: From Sumer to Saddam*, 3rd ed. New York: Palgrave Macmillan.

35 **to New Yorkers of 2001.:** Lifton, R.J. (1996). *Hiroshima in America.* New York: Harper Perennial.

36 **and other public policy entities:** Shlaes, A. (2007). *The forgotten man: A new history of the Great Depression.* New York: HarperCollins.

36 **and words of President Roosevelt:** Updike, J. *Laissez-faire is more: A revisionist history of the depression.* The New Yorker, July 02, 2007.

36 **his book *The Greatest Generation*:** Brokaw, T. (1998). *The greatest generation.* New York: Random House.

36 **explicit sexuality on the screen.:** Luke, C. (1990). *Constructing the child viewer: A history of the American discourse on television and children, 1950–1980.* New York: Praeger.

36 **viewer, including the child viewer.:** Hilmes, M. (2004). *The television history book.* London: British Film Institute.

37 **and faith in the future:** Garbarino, J. (2002). Foreword: pathways from childhood trauma to adolescent violence and delinquency. *Journal of Aggression, Maltreatment & Trauma* 6(1):22–29.

37 **"....finding meaning in your life?":** Vanderkolk, B. (1987). *Psychological trauma.* Washington, D.C.: American Psychiatric Press.

39 **the direction of universal coverage.:** Skocpol, T. (1997). *Boomerang: Health care reform and the turn against government.* New York: W.W. Norton & Company.

39 **more genrally fearful they are.:** Graber, D. (2005). *Mass media and American politics.* Washington, D.C.: CQ Press.

40 **answer is a clear "yes.":** Venables, R.W. (2004). *American Indian history: Five centuries of conflict & coexistence.* Santa Fe, NM: Clear Light Books.

40 **If you are were an African:** Genovese, E.D. (1988). *The political economy of slavery: Studies in the economy and society of the slave south.* Middletown, CT: Wesleyan University Press.

40 **If you are a suspected:** Mayer, J. *The Black Sites: A rare look inside the C.I.A.'s secret interrogation program.* The New Yorker, August 13, 2007.

40 **If you are convicted of:** Banner, S. (2003). *The death penalty: An American history.* Cambridge, MA: Harvard University Press.

40 **Magazine cover called them "monsters.":** Dickenson, A. *Where were the parents?* Time Magazine, May 03, 1999, 40.

40 **barbaric practice of executing minors.:** Tayor, G. *High court bans death row for minors.* The Washington Times, March 02, 2005.

40 **to a Yale University study.:** Lewin, T. *Research finds a high rate of expulsions in preschool.* The New York Times, May 17, 2005.

41 **had shrunk to about 20%.** Gruber, A. (2003). *Public finds government inefficient, study shows.* Available at govexec.com

41 **to only 16% in 1997).:** Hopkins, A. *U.S. families worry as families face deportation.* New York Times, August 29, 2007.

Chapter 4

43 **to be inappropriate and damaging.":** Garbarino, J., & Eckenrode, J. (1997). *Understanding abusive families.* San Francisco: Jossey-Bass.

44 **Indeed, Michael Rutter's recent review:** Rutter, M. (2007). Resilience, competence, and coping. *Child Abuse & Neglect* 31(3):205–209.

44 *violating the rights of others.*: American Psychiatric Association (2000). *Diagnostic and Statistical Manual of Mental Disorders DSM-IV-TR Fourth Edition.* Washington, D.C.: American Psychiatric Publishing.

44 **Kenneth Dodge and his colleagues:** Dodge, K.A., Petit, G.S., & Bates, J.E. (1997). How the experience of early physical abuse leads children to become chronically aggressive. In *Rochester Symposium on Developmental Psychopathology: Trauma: Perspectives on Theory, Research, and Intervention,* ed. D. Cicchetti and SL Toth. Rochester, NY: University of Rochester Press.

46 **Terrie Moffitt, and their colleagues.:** Caspi, A., McClay, J, Moffitt, T. et al. (2002). Evidence that the cycle of violence in maltreated children depends on genotype. *Science* 297:851–854.

46 **the research of Richard Tremblay):** Tremblay, R.E. (2000). The development of aggressive behavior during childhood. *International Journal of Behavioral Development* 24(2):129–141.

47 **by Tremblay, Tolan, and Guerra:** Tolan, P., & Guerra, N. (1998). *What works in reducing adolescent violence? An empirical review of the field.* Boulder, CO: Center for the Study and Prevention of Violence.

47 **seriously violent delinquents in adolescence.** Rutter, M. (1989). Pathways from childhood to adult life. *Journal of Child Psychology and Psychiatry* 30(1):23–51.

47 **David Olds and his colleagues:** Olds, D.L., Robinson, J., O'Brien, R., et al. (2002). Home visiting by paraprofessionals and by nurses: A randomized, controlled trial. *Pediatrics* 110(3):486–496.

47 **David Olds and his colleagues:** MacMillan, H.L., Jamieson, E., Walsh, C.A., et al. (2005). Effectiveness of home visitation by public-health nurses in prevention of the recurrence of child physical abuse and neglect: a randomised controlled trial. *Lancet* 365:1786–1793.

48 **neglected children do receive treatment:** Talley, P.F. (2005). *Handbook for treatment of abused and neglected children.* New York: Haworth Press.

52 **is told in his book:** Masters, J.J. (1997). *Finding freedom: Writings from death row.* Junction City, CA: Padma Publishing.

52 **report having witnessed a shooting.:** Bell, C., & Jenkins, E. (1993). Community violence and children on Chicago's southside. *Psychiatry* 56:46–54.

52 **West Bank and Gaza strip.:** Garbarino, J., & Kostelny, K. (1996). The effects of political violence on Palestinian children's behavior problems: A risk accumulation model. *Child Development* 67:33–45.

53 **civilized world considers this barbaric.:** Grisso, T. (1996). Society's retributive response to juvenile violence: A developmental perspective. *Law and Human Behavior* 20(3):229–247.

Chapter 5

55 **and attitudes that kids develop.:** Hess, R., & Torney, J. (2005). *Development of political attitudes in children.* Piscataway, NJ: Aldine Transaction.

55 **psychologist Urie Bronfenbrenner, and I.:** Garbarino, J., & Bronfenbrenner, U. (1976). The socialization and moral judgment and behavior in cross-cultural perspective. In T. Lickona (Ed.), *Moral development and behavior.* New York: Holt, Rinehart and Winston.

56 **by the research of Diana Baumrind:** Shaffer, D.B. (2006). *Developmental psychology,* 7th ed. Belmont, CA: Wadsworth.

57 **(such as sociologist Glen Elder:** Elder, G., Modell, J., & Parke, R. (1993) (eds.) *Children in time and place: Developmental and historical insights.* New York: Cambridge University Press.

57 **during the age of terror.:** Eldebour, S., Baker, A.M., & Charlesworth, W.R. (1997). The impact of political violence on moral reasoning in children. *Child Abuse & Neglect* 21(11):1053–1066.

57 **moral reasoning of their students.:** Fields, R. (1977). *Society under siege: A psychology of Northern Ireland.* Philadelphia: Temple University Press.

58 **widely on the national news.:** Norheimer, M. (2000, May 27). Seventh-grade boy held in killing of a teacher. New York Times. Retrieved June 2, 2006, from http://www.nytimes.com

59 **was likened, was also murdered:** Burns, J. (1998, March 2002). Hindu still proud of role in killing the father of India. New York Times. Retrieved June 2, 2006, from http://www.nytimes.com

61 **at Pearl Harbor in 1941.:** Daniels, R. (1993). *Prisoners without trial: Japanese Americans in World War II.* New York: Hill and Wang.

61 **earlier (from 40 to 269).:** BBC News (2005, August 2004). Hate crimes soar after bombings. Retrieved on May 18, 2007 from http://news.bbc.co.uk

62 **the war zone front lines.:** Garbarino, J. (1991) *No place to be a child: growing up in a war zone.* New York: Lexington Books.

62 **the political crisis is solved,:** Bettelheim, B. (1943). Individual and mass behavior in extreme situations. *Journal of Abnormal and Social Psychology* 38:417–452.

62 **through acts of violent revenge.:** Fields, R. (2004). *Martyrdom: The psychology, theology, and politics of self-sacrifice.* Westport, CT: Praeger Publishers.

62 **great psychiatrist Harry Stack Sullivan:** Sullivan, H.S. (1953). *The interpersonal theory of psychiatry.* New York: Norton.

63 **In *Children of the A-Bomb*:** Osada, A. (1982). *Children of the A-Bomb: Testament of the boys and girls of Hiroshima.* United States: Midwest Publishers International.

63 **revolting war we have now.:** Werner, E. (2001). *Through the eyes of innocents: Children witness World War II.* Boulder, CO: Westview Press.

63 **"Project Renewal Post 9/11":** Available at http://www.innerresilience-tidescenter.org

63 **Fellowship of Reconciliation:** Available at http://www.forusa.org

63 **The Nonviolence Web.:** Available at http://www.nonviolence.org

63 **and spiritual teacher Dave Richo.:** Richo, D. (1999). *Shadow dance.* Boston: Shambhala.

64 **Psychologist Scott Gibbs has conducted:** Gibbs, S. (2005). Islam and Islamic extremism: An existential analysis. *Journal of Humanistic Psychology* 45(2):156–203.

65 **(army) divisions does he command.":** Miner, S.M. (2007). *Stalin's holy war: Religion, nationalism, and alliance politics, 1941–1945.* Chapel Hill, NC: The University of North Carolina Press.

67 **says that violence is "demented.":** Gilligan, J. (1997). *Violence: Reflections on a national epidemic.* New York: Vintage Books.

Chapter 6

69 **other segments of the population.:** U.S. Bureau of the Census (2006). *Evaluation of poverty estimates: A comparison of the American community survey and the current population survey.* Census Bureau. Available at http://www.census.gov/hhes/www/poverty/acs_cpspovcompreport.pdf

70 **collect and report these data.:** Shah, A. (2006). *Causes of poverty.* Available at http://www.globalissues.org

70 **failure, maltreatment, and learning disabilities.:** Aber, J.L., & Bennett, N.G. (1997). The effects of poverty on child health and development. *Annual Review of Public Health* 18:463–483.

70 **like my mother's sibling.:** Mink, S.D. (1993). *Poverty, population, and the environment.* Washington, D.C.: World Bank.

70 **In Canada it has meant:** Battle, K. (1998). Transformation: Canadian social policy since 1985. *Social Policy & Administration* 32(4):321–340.

70 **United States than in Canada.:** Clement, M.E., & Bouchard, C. (2005). Predicting the use of single versus multiple types of violence towards children in a representative sample of Quebec families. *Child Abuse & Neglect* 29(10):1121–1139.

71 **according to Federal Government reports.:** Belix, W., & Grossi, M. (2003). *Brazil's zero hunger program in the context of social policy.* Presented at the 25th International Conference of Agricultural Economists, Durban, South Africa. Available at http://brazilbrazil.com/fome.html/

71 **Two world-renowned economists:** Sachs, J.D. (2005). *The end of poverty: Economic possibilities for our time.* New York: Penguin Press.

71 **Two world-renowned economists:** Yunus, M. (2003). *Banker to the poor: Micro-lending and the battle against world poverty.* New York: Public Affairs.

72 **"relative deprivation,":** Walker, I., & Pettigrew, T. F. (1984). Relative deprivation theory: an overview and conceptual critique. *British Journal of Social Psychology* 23:301–310.

73 **of the population are poor:** Blanc, L.S. (1994). *Urban children in distress.* London: Routledge.

73 **every society in the world.:** Garbarino, J. (1995). *Raising children in a socially toxic environment.* San Francisco: Jossey-Bass.

73 **every society in the world.:** Reppucci, D. (1983). *Emerging issues in the ecology of children and families.* Invited address to the 91st annual meeting, American Psychological Association, Anaheim, CA.

73 **every society in the world.:** Korbin, J. (1992). Introduction: Child poverty in the U.S. *The American Behavioral Scientist* 35:213–219.

73 **every society in the world.:** Bane, M., & Ellwood, D. (1989). *Slipping into and out of poverty: The dynamics of spells.* Cambridge, MA: National Bureau of Economic Research.

73 **every society in the world.:** Garbarino, J. (1992). The meaning of poverty to children. *American Behavioral Scientist* 35:220–237.

74 **conducted in the non-monetarized economy.:** Garbarino, J. (1992). *Towards a sustainable society.* Chicago: The Noble Press; and http://www.timebanks.org

75 **the United Nations Development Program:** United Nations. *Human development report 1999: Globalization with a human face.* New York.

75 **The Luxembourg Income Study:** *Luxembourg income study.* Available at http://www.lis-project.org/

76 **this inequality is the Gini Index.:** Corporate Watch (1997). *The Corporate Planet.* Available at http://www.corpwatch.org/

76 **particularly health and nutritional needs.:** Kochanek, K.D., & Martin, J.A. (2007). *Supplemental analyses of recent trends in infant mortality.* National Center for Health Statistics. Available at http://www.cdc.gov/nchs/products/pubs/pubd/hestats/infantmort/infantmort.htm

76 **provision of maternal-infant care.:** Brosco, J. (1999). The early history of the infant mortality rate in America. *Pediatrics* 103(2):478–488.

76 **hardest hit by economic disintegration.:** Garbarino, J. (1992). The meaning of poverty in the world of children. *American Behavioral Scientist*, 35:220–237.

76 **institutions such as the World Bank.:** Shah, A. (2007). *Structural adjustment: A major cause of poverty.* Available at http://www.globalissues.org

77 **social conditions were extremely harsh.:** Hewlett, S.A. (1980). *Cruel dilemmas of development: Twentieth-century Brazil.* New York: Basic Books.

77 ***The Nation* magazine, Marc Cooper:** Cooper, M. (2002). *Pinochet and me: A Chilean anti-memoir.* New York: Verso.

78 **a massive bio-fuels program.:** Morgan, D. (2005, June 18). Brazil's biofuel strategy pays off as gas prices soar. Washington Post. Retrieved on June 02, 2006, from http://www.washingtonpost.com

78 **enormous income inequalities in Brazil:** ReVista: Harvard review of Latin America (2007). *Brazil the search for equity.*

78 **were considered "abandoned" by UNICEF.:** Williams, R. (1987). *UNICEF "Children and World Development.* London: Richmond Publishing.

78 **his history of *The Soviet Family.*:** Geiger, H.K. (1968). *The family in Soviet Russia.* Cambridge, MA: Harvard University Press.

78 **his history of *The Soviet Family.*:** Avtonomov, V.S., Kuznetsov, A.P., Mitskevitch, A.A., Sheram, K.A., & Soubbotina, T.P. (1999). *The world and Russia.* St. Petersburg, Russia: World Bank Institute.

80 **educator-psychologist A. S. Makarenko:** Makarenko, A.S. (1967). *The collective family.* New York: Doubleday.

82 **28 per 1000 in 2007:** Assis, M. (2006). *Brazil reduces infant mortality to 24 deaths per 1000.* Brazil Magazine.

Chapter 7

83 **For example, the World Health:** *World Report on Violence and Health (2002).* World Health Organization. Available at http://www.who.int/violence_injury_prevention/violence/world_report/en/full_en.pdf

84 **According to her autobiography, *Blackberry Winter*,:** Mead, M. (1989). *Blackberry winter: My earlier years.* New York: Peter Smith Publishing.

85 **any means in the United States.:** Tierney, K.J. (1982). The battered wife movement and the creation of the wife beating problem. *Social Problems* 29:207–220.

85 **As psychologist Emmy Werner:** Werner, E. (2000). Protective factors and individual resilience, in Shonkoff, J., & Meisels, S. (eds.), *The Handbook of Early Interventions.* Cambridge University Press, New York.

85 **as culture and society change.:** Tolan, P., & Guerra, N. (1998). *What works in reducing adolescent violence? An empirical review of the field.* Boulder, CO: Center for the Study and Prevention of Violence.

85 **entering college at higher rates,:** Chaplin, D., & Klasik, D. (2006). *Gender gaps in college and high school graduation rates by race, combining public and private schools.* Available at http://www.uark.edu/ua/der/EWPA/Research/Accountability/1790.html

86 **thus androgyny increases for females:** Life Expectancy Hits Record High: Gender Gap Narrows. National Center for Health Statistics. Available at www.cdc.gov/nchs/pressroom/05facts/lifeexpectancy.htm

86 **As anthropologist Ronald Rohner documented:** Rohner, R.P. (1975). *They love me, they love me not: A worldwide study of the effects of parental acceptance and rejection.* New Haven, CT: Human Relations Area Files.

86 **disrupts development and distorts behavior.:** Downey, G., Irwin, L., Ramsay, M., & Ozlem, A. (2004). Rejection sensitivity and girls aggression, in Moretti, M.M., Jackson, M.A., & Odgers, C.L. (eds.), *Girls and aggression: Contributing factors and intervention principles.* New York: Kluwer Academic/Plenum.

87 **repatriated to the United States.:** Bixler, M. (2006). *The lost boys of Sudan: An American story of the refugee experience.* Athens, GA: The University of Georgia Press.

87 **"International Foster Parent Plan":** Available at http://www.plan-international.org/

87 **(not statistically surprising in a...:** Available at http://indexmundi.com

87 **size of pin hole.:** United States State Department (2001). *Sudan: Report on female genital mutilation (FGM) or female genital cutting (FGC).* Available at http://www.state.gov/g/wi/rls/rep/crfgm/10110.htm

88 **the capacity for sexual gratification:** World Health Organization. (1995). *Female genital mutilation: Report of a WHO Technical Working Group.* Geneva: World Health Organization.

88 ***Women Why Do You Weep?:*** El Dareer, A. (1982). *Women, why do you weep?* London: Zed Press.

89 **challenged and stopped in China.:** Wang, P., & Ping, W. (2000). *Aching for beauty: Footbinding in China.* Minneapolis: University of Minnesota Press.

90 **cultural differences in human development.:** Garbarino, J., & Ebata, A. (1983). The significance of ethnic and cultural differences in child maltreatment. *Journal of Marriage and the Family* 45(4):773–783.

90 **Swiss psychoanalyst Alice Miller:** Miller, A. (1991). *Thou shalt not be aware: Society's betrayal of the child.* New Haven, CT: Meridian Books.

Chapter 8

93 **have to take you in.—:** Frost, R. (2002). *Robert Frost's poems.* New York: St. Martin's Press.

93 **"attachment" is the first such map.:** Shaffer, D.B. (2006). *Developmental psychology,* 7th ed. Belmont, CA: Wadsworth.

93 **their attachment maps early on,:** Cassidy, J., & Shaver, P.R. (1999). *Handbook of attachment: Theory, research, and clinical applications.* New York: The Guilford Press.

94 **The psychoanalyst Erik Erikson:** Erikson, E.H. (1995). *Childhood and society.* New York: Vintage.

94 **to have disrupted attachment relationships.:** Holland, R., Kimberly, D., & Moretti, M.M. (2004). Aggression from an attachment perspective, in Jackson, M.A., Moretti, M.M., & Odgers, C.L. (eds.), *Girls and aggression: Contributing factors and intervention principles.* New York: Kluwer Academic/Plenum.

94 **H. L. Mencken offered an:** Mencken, H.L. (1926). *Prejudices.* New York: Alfred A. Knopf.

96 **child's right to cultural identity.:** Bartholet, E. (1991). Where do Black children belong? The politics of race matching in adoption. *University of Pennsylvania Law Review* 139(5):1163–1256.

96 **Tibetan cultural identity in exile.:** Servan-Schreiber, D., Lin, B., & Birmaher, B. (1998). Prevalence of posttraumatic stress disorder and major depressive disorder in Tibetan refugee children. *Journal of American Academy of Child and Adolescent Psychiatry* 37(8):874–879.

96 **identity become salient and insistent.:** Phinney, J.S. (1990). Ethnic identity in adolescents and adults: review of research. *Psychological Bulletin* 108(3):499–514.

97 **is likely to be disastrous.:** Kim, W.J. (1995). International adoption: a case review of Korean children. *Child Psychiatry and Human Development* 25(3):141–154.

97 **cultural disconnection as an adolescent).:** Doyle, A., & Moretti, M. (2002). *Attachment to parents and adjustment in adolescence.* Ottawa, Canada. Division of Childhood and Adolescence, Public Health Agency of Canada.

97 **I find historian Amy Kaplan's:** Kaplan, A. (2003). Homeland insecurities: Reflections on language and space. *Radical History Review* 85:82–93.

97 **the efforts of the citizenry.:** The White House (2001). *Gov. Ridge Sworn-In to Lead Homeland Security.* Available at http://www.whitehouse.gov/news/releases/2001/10/20011008-3.html

98 **the experience of family disintegration.:** Kelly, J.B. (2000). Children's adjustment in conflicted marriage and divorce: a decade review of research. *Journal of the American Academy of Child and Adolescent Psychiatry* 39(8):963–973.

98 **and competence to their children.:** Garbarino, J. (1995). The American war zone. *Journal of Developmental and Behavioral Pediatrics* 16:431–435.

98 **and competence to their children.:** Garbarino, J., & Vorrasi, J. (1999). Long term effects of war on children. *Encyclopedia of Violence, Peace, and Conflict* 2:345–359.

98 **book *Everything in its Path*,:** Erikson, K.T. (1978). *Everything in its path: Destruction of community in the Buffalo Creek Flood.* New York: Touchstone.

98 **includes school, neighbourhood, and friends.:** Bronfenbrenner, U. (2006). *The ecology of human development: Experiments by nature and design.* Cambridge, MA: Harvard University Press.

99 **children think in concrete terms,:** Shaffer, D.B. (2006). *Developmental psychology*, 7th ed. Belmont, CA: Wadsworth.

99 **importance of identity in adolescence.:** Kroger, J. (2005). *Identity in adolescence: The balance between self and other.* New York: Routledge.

99 **Erik Erikson went so far:** Erikson, E.H. (1994). *Identity and the life cycle.* New York: Norton.

100 **government in the 18th century,:** Ryerson, R., & Fremont-Barnes, G. (2006). *The encyclopedia of the American revolutionary war: A political, social, and military history.* New York: ABC-CLIO.

100 **Arab rivals for the territory).:** Zadka, S. (2003). *Blood in Zion: How the Jewish guerrillas drove the British out of Palestine.* London: Brassey's.

100 **Organization to coordinate their struggle).:** Carter, J. (2007). *Palestine peace not apartheid.* New York: Simon & Schuster.

100 **known as the Gaza Strip.:** Bennis, P. (2007). *Understanding the Palestinian-Israeli conflict: A primer.* New York: Olive Branch Press.

101 **we are, a sovereign state.":** Available at http://www.ajc.org

101 **them in the 19th century.:** New York Times (1983, Dec. 11). Plan to settle Cayugas' land claim weighed. Retrieved on July 27, 2006, from http://www.newyorktimes.com

101 **integrity of their homeland territory.:** Vandervort, B. (2006). *Indian Wars of Canada, Mexico and the United States: 1812–1900.* New York: Routledge.

104 **of America's economically displaced persons:** Garbarino, J., Dubrow, N., Kostelny, K., & Pardo, C. (1998). *Children in danger: Coping with the consequences of community violence.* San Francisco: Jossey-Bass.

105 ***Voices from the Camps: Vietnamese Children Seeking Assylum.*:** Freeman, J.M., & Huu, N.D. (2003). *Voices from the camps: Vietnamese children seeking asylum.* Seattle: University of Washington Press.

105 **focus on the day-to-day.:** Defrancisci, L., Lubit, R., Rovine, D., & Spencer, E.T. (2003). Impact of trauma on children. *Journal of Psychiatric Practice* 9(2):128–138.

Chapter 9

107 **from Dostoyevsky's *The Brothers Karamazov:*** Dostoyevsky, F. (1900). *The brothers Karamazov.* New York: Barnes and Noble Books.

107 **peace, peace is the way.":** Hanh, T.N. (2005). *Being peace.* Berkeley, CA: Parallax Press.

107 **to see in the world.":** Fisher, L., Gandhi, Gandhi, M., & Gandhi, M.K. (2002). *The essential Gandhi: An anthology of his writings on his life, work, and ideas.* New York: Vintage.

108 **differentiate between civilians and combatants.:** Van Creveld, M. (2007). *The changing face of war: Lessons of combat, from the Marne to Iraq.* New York: Presidio Press.

108 **half of those are children.:** UNICEF (n.d.). Children in Conflict and Emergencies. Available at http://www.unicef.org/protection/index_armedconflict.html

108 **never do just one thing.":** Harden, G. (1995). *Living within limits: Ecology, economics, and population taboos.* New York: Oxford University Press.

108 **vaccine on the immune system.:** Cave, S., & Mitchell, D. (2001). *What your doctor may not tell you about children's vaccinations.* New York: Grand Central Publishing.

108 **is segregation by social class.:** Deenesh, S., & Salvatore, S. (2007). Mapping educational inequality: Concentrations of poverty among poor and minority students in public schools. *Social Forces* 85(3):1227–1253.

108 **simmers between Sunnis and Shittes.:** Galbraith, P.W. (2007). *The end of Iraq: How American incompetence created a war without end.* New York: Simon & Schuster.

109 ***Children Witness World War II.*:** Werner, E.E. (2001). *Through the eyes of innocents: Children witness World War II.* Boulder, CO: Westview Press.

109 **of Allied Coalition forces.:** Leavitt, L., & Fox, N. (1993). *The psychological effects of war and violence on children.* Mahwah, NJ: Lawrence Erlbaum and Associates.

110 **with European and Japanese losses.:** The National WWII Museum. *World War II By The Numbers.* Available at http://www.ddaymuseum.org/education/education_numbers.html

110 **death total in American history.:** Reed, C. (2004). *A minor event in terms of war casualties worldwide.* Available at www.counterpunch.org

111 **for reasons of "national security.":** Kashima, T. (2003). *Judgment without trial: Japanese American imprisonment during World War II.* Seattle, WA: University of Washington Press.

111 **in executing this odious mission.:** Houston, J.D., & Houston, J.W. (1983). *Farewell to Manzanar: A true story of Japanese American experience during and after the World War II internment.* New York: Bantam Books.

112 **the social realities they face.:** Garbarino, J., & Manley, J. (1996). Free and captured play: Releasing the healing power. *International Play Journal* 4:123–132.

112 **War II it was 50%.:** Apfel, R., & Simon, B. (1996). *Minefields in their hearts.* New Haven, CT: Yale University Press.

113 **and infrastructure of the South.:** Neely, M. (2004). *Was the Civil War a total war?* Retrieved on September 22, 2006, from http://muse.jhu.edu/journals/civil_war_history/v050/50.4neely.html

113 **conducted to answer this question.:** Heath, A., Ryan, K., Dean, B., & Bingham, R. (2007). *History of school safety and psychological first aid for children. Brief Treatment and Crisis Intervention.* 7:206–223.

113 **Canadian pediatrician Susan Goldberg:** Goldberg, S., LaCombe, S.L., Levinson, D., Ross, C., & Sommers, F.G. (1986). Children in fear of nuclear war. *World Health Forum* 7(4):399–401.

114 **Kahn's book *On Thermonuclear War.*:** Kahn, H. (1960). *The thermonuclear war.* Princeton, NJ: Princeton University Press.

114 ***The Fate of the Earth,*:** Schell, J. (1982). *The fate of the earth.* New York: Knopf.

114 **figure had grown to 35%.:** Beardslee, W.R., Goodman, L.A., Mack, J.E., & Snow, R.M. (1983). The threat of nuclear war and the nuclear arms race: Adolescent experience and perceptions. *Political Psychology* 4(3):501–530.

114 **decades of the nuclear age.:** Ptacek, C (1988). The nuclear age: Context for family interaction. *Family Relations* 37(4):337–343.

114 **increased pessimism about the future.:** Fiske, S.T., & Schatz, R.T. (1992). International reactions to the threat of nuclear war: The rise and fall of concern in the eighties. *Political Psychology* 13(1):1–29.

115 **such as low energy levels.:** Aiko, S. (2004). Surviving Hiroshima and Nagasaki: Experiences and psychosocial meanings. *Psychiatry* 67:43–62.

115 **was not linked to pessimism.:** Achenbach Child Behavior Check List data. Available at http://www.aseba.org

115 **of this deployment on children.:** Henderson, K. (2006). *While they're at war: The true story of American families on the homefront.* New York: Mariner Books.

115 **the fighting in Iraq alone.:** Available at http://www.usakia.org

115 **families—and thus children.:** *Children and the news: Coping with terrorism, war and everyday violence.* Key facts, Spring 2003. Menlo Park, CA: The Henry Kaiser Family Foundation.

116 **psychological effects of war trauma.:** Global attitudes project. Philadelphia: Pew Research Center. Available at http://www.pewglobal.org

116 **virulent anti-American education programs.:** Sennott, C.M. (2002). *Saudi schools fuel anti-US anger.* Boston Globe.

116 **girls started attending school:** Reynolds, M. (2005). Afghan girls go to school—Slowly, surely. Fox News. Retrieved on September 25, 2006. Available at http://www.foxnews.com

116 **democratic society might look like.:** Ghosh, B. (2005, February 07). A vote for hope. Time. Retrieved on September 25, 2006. Available at http://www.time.com

117 **and waning of terrorist campaigns.:** Costello, J., Masten, A., & Pine, D.S. (2005). Trauma, proximity, and developmental psychopathology: The effects of war and terrorism on children. *Neuropsychopharmacology* 30:1781–1792.

117 **economic situation…was satisfactory.":** Carter, J.C. (2006). *Palestine: Peace not apartheid.* New York: Simon & Schuster.

117 **they knew a person killed.:** Solomon, Z., & Laufer, A. (2004). In the shadow of terror: Changes in world assumptions in Israeli youth. *Journal of Aggression, Maltreatment and Trauma* 9:353–364.

118 **of any one risk factor.:** Bedard, C. (2007). *Children's rights are human rights.* Chicago: Loyola University Press, Center for the Human Rights of Children.

118 **wounded or died in war.":** Klingman, A., Sagi, A., & Raviv, A. (1993). The effect of war on Israeli children. In L.A. Leavitt and N.A. Fox (eds.), *Psychological effects of war and violence on children.* Hillsdale, NJ: Lawrence Erlbaum Associates.

118 **fifth and sixth grade children.:** Milgram, R. M., & Milgram, N. A. (1976). The effect of the Yom Kippur War on anxiety level in Israeli children. *Journal of Psychology* 94:107–113.

118 **A study of Israeli children:** Ziv, A., & Israeli, R. (1973), Effects of bombardment on the manifest anxiety level of children living in kibbutzim. *Journal of Consulting and Clinical Psychology* 40:287–291.

119 **The more religious Israeli youth:** Weaver, A. J., Flannely, L. T., Flannely, K. J., Koenig, H. G., & Larson, D. B. (1998). An analysis of research on religions and spiritual variables in three major mental health nursing journals. *Issues in Mental Health Journals* 19:263–276.

119 **American research reveals the same:** Miller, L., Davies, M., & Greenwaled, S. (2000). Religiosity and substance use and abuse among adolescents in the National Comorbidity Survey. *American Academy of Child and Adolescent Psychiatry* 39(9):1190–1197.

119 **than their more secular counterparts.:** Hyde, K. (1990). *Religion in childhood and adolescence.* Birmingham, AL: Religion Education Press.

119 **Israeli researchers Zahava Solomon:** Solomon, Z., & Laufer, A. (2005). In the shadow of terror: Changes in world assumptions in Israeli youth. *Journal of Aggression Maltreatment and Trauma* 9(3):353–364.

119 **psychologist Charles Greenbaum and his:** Greenbaum, C.W., Veerman, P., & Bacon-Shnoor, N. (2006). *Protection of children during armed political conflict.* Schoten, Belgium: Intersentia Publishers.

120 **When I read Moses' analysis:** Moses, R. (1982). The group self and the Arab-Israeli conflict. *The International Review of Psychoanalysis* 9:55–64.

120 **violent neighborhoods in America.:** Garbarino, J. (1999). *Lost boys: Why our sons turn violent and how we can save them.* New York: Anchor.

120 **endeavor shrink to insignificance.":** Farago, L. (1963). *Ordeal and triumph.* New York: Ivan Obolensky.

120 **"The Moral Equivalent to War":** James, W. (1971). *The moral equivalent of war, and other essays: And selections from some problems of philosophy.* New York: Harper & Row.

Chapter 10

123 **dispute the passage with you?":** Anonymous.

123 **struggle, sadness, and disappointment).:** Mullen, S.J. (1914). *The spiritual exercises of St. Ignatius of Loyola.* New York: PJ Kennedy & Sons.

123 **Buddhism teaches that suffering is:** Hanh, T.N. (2003). *Opening the heart of the cosmos: Insights on the Lotus Sutra.* Berkeley, CA: Parallax Press.

123 **is from moment to moment,":** Hahn, T.N. (1999). *The miracle of mindfulness.* New York: Bantam.

124 **"The Therapy of Reassurance.":** Garbarino, J. (2001). An ecological perspective on the effects of violence on children. *Journal of Community Psychology* 29(3):361–378.

124 **posttraumatic stress disorder diagnosis.:** Schlenger, W. (2002). Psychological reactions to terrorist attacks. *Journal of the American Medical Association* 288:581–588.

124 **crisis situations around the world.:** Boothby, N., Ressler, E.M., & Steinbock, D.J. (1988). *Unaccompanied children: Care and protection in wars, natural disasters and refugee movements.* New York: Oxford University Press.

124 **return to emotional equilibrium.:** Faust, J., & Gold, S.N. (2003). *Trauma practice in the wake of September 11, 2001.* Binghamton, NY: Haworth Maltreatment and Trauma Press.

125 **Psychologist George Bonanno:** Bonanno, G.A. (2004). Loss, trauma, and human resilience: Have we underestimated the human capacity to thrive after extremely aversive events? *American Psychologist* 59:20–28.

125 **stability, and security.:** Pynoos, R., & Eth, S. (1985). Developmental perspectives on psychic trauma in childhood. In Figley R., ed. *Trauma and its wake.* New York: Brunner/Mazel.

125 **need professional mental health services.:** Achenbach, T.M., & Howell, C.T. (1993). Are American children's problems getting worse? A 13-year comparison. *Journal of American Academy of Child and Adolescent Psychiatry* 32(6):1145–1154.

126 **For example, during the Gulf:** Dubrow N., Garbarino J., & Kostelny, K. (1991). What children can tell us about living in danger. *American Psychologist* 46:376–383.

126 **In Burstow's terms:** Burstow, B. (2005). A critique of posttraumatic stress disorder and the DSM. *Journal of Humanistic Psychology* 45(4):429–445.

127 **struggling prior to 9/11.:** Schlenger, W. (2002). Psychological reactions to terrorist attacks. *Journal of the American Medical Association* 288:581–588.

127 **child's own direct exposure.:** Hoven, C.W., Duarte, C. S., Lucas, C. P., Mandell, D. J., & Co. *Effects of the World Trade Center attack on NYC public school students: Initial report to the board of education.* Prepared by Applied Research and Consulting, LLC (New York), the Columbia University Mailman School of Public Health, and the New York State Psychiatric Institute, May 6, 2002.

127 **Among the specific procedures:** Shapiro, F. (2001). *Eye movement desensitization and reprocessing (EMDR),* 2nd ed. *Basic Principles, Protocols, and Procedures.* New York: Guilford Press.

127 **However, there is nothing:** Carbonell, J.L., & Figley, C.R. (1999). Running head: Promising PTSD treatment approaches. *Traumatology* 5:32–48.

128 **the child to future separations.:** Silver, R.C., Holman, E.A., McIntosh, D.N., Poulin, M., & Gil-Rivas, V. (2002). Nationwide longitudinal study of psychological responses to September 11. *Journal of the American Medical Association* 288:1235–1244.

128 **exposure to cause and effect.:** Kramer, P.D. (1998). Listening to Prozac: A psychiatrist explores antidepressant drugs and the remaking of the self. Darby, PA: DIANE Publishing.

128 **standing trial for murder.:** Garbarino, J. (1999). *Lost boys: Why our sons turn violent and how we can save them.* New York: Anchor.

128 **The answer was, "98%.":** Grossman, D. (1996). *On killing: The psychological cost of learning to kill in war and society.* Boston: Back Bay Books.

129 **of their horrible experience?:** Perry, B.D., & Szalavitz, M. (2007). *The boy who was raised as a dog: And other stories from a child psychiatrist's notebook: What traumatized children can teach us about loss, love and healing.* Cambridge, MA: Basic Books.

129 **brain functions when aroused.:** Perry, B.D., Pollard, R.A., Blakley, T.L., Baker, D., & Viglante, D. (1995). Childhood trauma, the neurobiology of adaptation, and "use-dependent" development of the brain: How "states" become "traits." *Infant Mental Health Journal* 16(4):271–291.

131 **warm and supportive families.:** Garbarino, J., & Kostelny, K. (1996). The effects of political violence on Palestinian children's behavior problems: a risk accumulation model. *Child Development* 67:33–45.

132 **produce emotionally healthy children.:** Garbarino, J., & Bedard, C. (2001). *Parents under siege: Why you are the solution, not the problem, in your child's life.* New York: The Free Press.

Epilogue

135 **problem-neat, plausible and wrong.":** Mencken, H.L. (1920). *Prejudices*, 2nd series. Available at http://www.quotationspage.com

Index

Printed in the United States